Nourishing Motherhood

A Comprehensive Guide to Postnatal Vitamins, Remedies, and Recipes

Steven O. Forte

Nourishing Motherhood

Copyright

Every right reserved. With the exception of brief quotations included in critical reviews and certain other noncommercial uses allowed by copyright law, no part of this publication may be copied, distributed, or transmitted in any way or by any means, including photocopying, recording, or other electronic or mechanical methods, without the publisher's prior written consent.

Steven O. Forte, Copyright © 2024.

Disclaimer

The material on this platform is intended for general informative purposes only. While we make every effort to keep the information accurate and up to date, we make no express or implied representations or warranties about the completeness, accuracy, reliability, suitability, or availability of the platform's information, products, services, or related graphics for any purpose. You assume all risks associated with relying on such material.

In no circumstances will Steven O. Forte be liable for any loss or harm, including but not limited to indirect or consequential loss or damage, or any loss or damage whatsoever resulting from data or profit loss deriving from, or in connection with, the use of this platform.

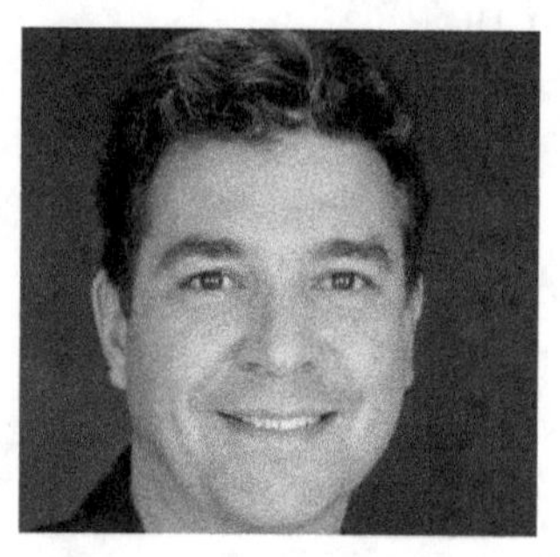

About the author

Steven O. Forte combines his knowledge of nutrition, wellness, and human experience to become an enthusiastic supporter of holistic well-being. Steven, who has experience as a nutritionist, offers a distinct viewpoint on the postpartum experience and highlights the significance of a holistic approach to health.

Utilizing a wealth of knowledge and a strong dedication to advancing wellbeing. His approach is motivated by his conviction that postpartum empowerment may be achieved through mindful practices, a supportive environment, and a balanced diet.

As a Certified Nutritionist, Steven is committed to offering readers evidence-based knowledge and useful ideas to help them navigate the complex world of postnatal health. His writing is kind, sympathetic, and based on a sincere appreciation of the pleasures and difficulties of motherhood.

The goal of Steven O. Forte is to empower people on their wellness journeys by reducing the complexity of health ideas and making them useful in day-to-day living. By his writings, he hopes to encourage readers to adopt a comprehensive perspective on postpartum health and support a robust and successful transition into this life-changing stage.

TABLE OF CONTENTS

INTRODUCTION

The postnatal period is a special time in the amazing adventure of motherhood, one that requires close attention to the growth of the new mother as well as her priceless bundle of joy. This all-inclusive guide is meant to be your friend; it offers insights into the fundamentals of postpartum nutrition, natural cures for common diseases, and a wonderful selection of dishes that feed the body and the spirit.

This guide goes beyond the commonplace as we explore the complex world of postpartum health, exploring the depths of vital minerals like vitamin D, iron, and B vitamins. We examine their enormous effects on immunity, energy, and general health, piecing together the complex picture of postnatal health.

Learn about natural cures for common postpartum illnesses, providing you with easy-to-use options. This comprehensive book tackles a range of issues, including weariness and mood swings, by stressing the use of natural solutions into your everyday routine.

With the help of our carefully chosen assortment of dishes, you may excite your taste buds and add vital nutrients to your diet while going on a gourmet adventure. These dishes, which range from meals high in iron to treats high in Omega-3 fatty acids that promote cognitive function, are made to make eating well a joyful part of your everyday routine.

We help you choose the best postnatal vitamin supplement by navigating the options available. Understanding labels, formulas, and specific demands are important because they help you make decisions that are specific to your own health needs.

Beyond diet, we explore holistic approaches to wellness, including mindfulness, self-care routines, relaxation methods, and activities appropriate for recently arrived mothers. This adventure ends with a fast-reference guide that simplifies important information for rapid access and gives you power while you're on the go.

As you immerse yourself in "Nourishing Motherhood," may it serve as your dependable guide, pointing the way toward a postpartum experience that is incredibly nourishing on many fronts in addition to being lively and healthy. Accept this journey with assurance, knowing that you have the skills and information necessary to support a vibrant and successful motherhood.

establishing the conditions for postpartum health. Creating a welcoming and encouraging atmosphere for new mothers as they embark on this special journey in their life is analogous to setting the stage for postnatal well-being. Think of it as the play's first act, where we recognize the difficulties and rewards associated with being a mother.

In this environment, we notice significant changes occurring not just in the physical realm but also in the emotional and mental domains. We want to make sure that this transition is as easy and supportive as we can during this period of change.

Imagine the idea that self-care is a necessity rather than a nice-to-have shown on the stage. We advise new mothers to prioritize self-care, be gentle to themselves, and take those breaks. We want to create an environment where health is a journey rather than a goal.

In the middle of the difficulties, nutrition is highlighted. We are speaking of the excellent stuff, the postnatal vitamins that turn into bodily replenishers and supporters of the needs of nursing, like superheroes. Not only should the tank be filled, but the emotional and mental resilience should also be nourished.

Creating an environment where mothers feel heard and understood is another way to set the groundwork for postnatal well-being. Here, we all value candid communication. Every woman has a distinct journey, and we value this variety. We're creating a community where people connect, exchange experiences, and find assistance.

This is not a production that is meant for everyone. Because the script is adaptable, it may be customized to meet the needs and tastes of any individual. It's a call to take an active role in one's health and acknowledge that self-care is an essential component of a happy and healthy postpartum experience rather than a luxury.

Imagine therefore that as we create the scene, it will be one of understanding, compassion, and celebration of the amazing adventure that is motherhood. May the entire health of the mother and child be highlighted as the curtains rise, telling a story that is both empowering and nurturing.

Establishing a warm, welcoming environment that helps new mothers feel supported and understood as they take on the role of parenting is one way to set the foundation for postnatal well-being. This location serves as the play's opening scene, a story that begins with the recognition of the highs and lows that characterize the postpartum experience.

We recognize that, in this cozy setting, this is a period of both physical and emotional transformation. The goal of setting the stage is to make this shift soothing and soft, to act as a calming background that helps new mothers adjust to the significant changes they are going through.

Imagine the idea that self-care is a need rather than a luxury shown on the stage. Moms are encouraged to prioritize relaxation, take time for themselves, and embrace self-care because of the gentle lighting. The environment is created with the intention of making well-being a continuous process rather than a destination, enabling moms to flourish.

The focus is on nourishment amidst the difficulties, particularly those super powerful postnatal vitamins. These nutrients play the role of supporting actors, providing the body with the necessary nourishment as well as the emotional and mental fortitude needed during this period of transformation. It's similar to giving the soul a filling supper.

Facilitating a conversation and a shared experience is another way to set the stage for postnatal well-being. Every woman's path is respected and honored in this place. It is now possible to have candid discussions, offer support to one another, and form bonds with other women who share the particular difficulties at this time.

This is a flexible production, not a stiff performance. The script is customizable, acknowledging that every mother has particular requirements and preferences. It's a call to action to take charge of one's health and realize that self-care is essential to a happy and healthy postpartum experience.

Imagine a world full of understanding, compassion, and a celebration of the amazing adventure that is motherhood as we continue to set the stage. Let the spotlight shine on the strength and resiliency that make this journey uplifting and immensely nourishing for both mother and child, as well as the challenges, when the curtains rise.

highlighting how crucial it is to approach nutrition and health from a holistic perspective. Consider viewing your well-being as more than just a meal plan. Stressing the significance of a comprehensive strategy for nutrition and well-being is akin to saying, "Hey, let's take a look at this big picture here." It's important to realize that being healthy involves a variety of factors rather than becoming fixated on calories or reaching dietary targets.

Consider it as caring for your well-being from the inside out. It's important to nourish your soul in addition to your body. Food becomes a source of happiness, coziness, and connection rather than just fuel. Your attitude, energy level, and general well-being are all impacted by the food you consume. It goes beyond only your physical well-being.

Imagine now a concentration on equilibrium. It has nothing to do with rigid diet plans or feeling bad about indulging in your guilty pleasure. It's about learning to appreciate a range of cuisines, engaging in mindful eating, and understanding that your decisions affect more than just your physical well-being. It's an eating style that fosters a positive relationship with food without being constrained by restrictions or guilt.

This comprehensive approach encompasses not only what's on your plate but also your way of life. Realizing that a healthy diet is only one piece of the jigsaw is important. A healthy lifestyle includes stress management, regular exercise, and restful sleep. It's realizing that self-care involves a variety of approaches that all add to your general state of health.

From this angle, your health is a dynamic entity. It's linked and dynamic, much like taking care of a garden. To build a life that is bright and growing, you tend to the soil (nutrition), ensure that there is enough sunlight (exercise), and control the weeds (stress).

Empowerment is at the center of it all. It's about arming you with the information and resources you need to make decisions that promote your wellbeing. Imagine a journey in which you are cultivating a sense of harmony that permeates every aspect of your life, in addition to providing nourishment for your body. The allure of a holistic approach lies in its emphasis on internal and external well-being.

CHAPTER 1:
Understanding Postnatal Nutrition

Mastering postnatal nutrition is like getting access to a secret recipe book made just for the amazing journey of motherhood. It's a voyage into the core of nourishment designed specifically for this special stage of life, not simply about what's on your plate.

Think of it as a helpful companion guiding new mothers through the challenges of feeding both themselves and their infants. It all comes down to realizing how important postnatal nutrition is to the healing process and meeting the needs of nursing while also assisting the body in mending.

We recognize the heroic alterations a woman's body experiences following childbirth in this view. It's more than just adding more nutrients—it's more akin to a restorative endeavor. Important factors that support immunity, energy levels, and general vigor come to the fore. These include crucial vitamins and minerals.

Consider postpartum nutrition as a roadmap for your unique journey. Since every mom's journey is different, the emphasis is on adjusting nutrient intake to meet specific needs. It's about choosing decisions that align with your personal health and well-being, taking into account things like nursing, lifestyle, and particular medical needs.

See it as a celebration of different meals that support healthy nutrition throughout pregnancy. The stage is set for a varied and fulfilling diet, with everything from protein-rich treats and nutritious grains to vibrant fruits and vegetables. Achieving nutritional objectives is not the only goal; enjoying a diverse range of tastes that makes self-nourishment enjoyable is also important.

From this perspective, postnatal nutrition is not a band-aid solution. It all comes down to creating enduring behaviors that promote long-term health. The emphasis is on building resilience and energy in mothers as they embrace the wonderful complexities of parenthood, and on laying the groundwork for continued well-being.

Knowing postnatal nutrition is ultimately about taking control of your health. It's about being informed enough to make decisions that support your child's growth and development in addition to providing nourishment for your own body. Imagine a journey where food becomes a source of resiliency, joy, and strength, illustrating the vibrant and blooming nature of the postnatal experience.

A postnatal diet that is precisely specified is essential for a new mother's overall health. A woman's body need a postnatal diet to recuperate from the weariness of pregnancy and childbirth. Making sure the woman is well hydrated is the first step towards her recovery. The body is weak and the digestive system cannot operate at its peak during the postpartum period. As a result, drinking water facilitates digestion and is required for producing enough breast milk. Nutrient- and vitamin-rich foods are essential components of this kind of diet. Consuming vegetables like spinach, carrots, and gourds is advised.

Foods heavy in lipids or carbs are essential for maintaining energy levels. Avoiding junk food is advised at all costs. Eat a place of dry fruits like raisins and cashews. There are plenty of options in an Indian cuisine to meet the demands of a nursing mother. Lentils or dal give the body the proteins it needs to fight infection. A balanced amount of clarified butter is used to make laddoos, which offer fats, while gond or tree gum improves lactation. Grains of any kind, including rice and wheat, are beneficial to health. In addition to this, chia and fenugreek seeds facilitate easy lactation.

Investigating the particular dietary requirements of nursing mothers.

Nutrition for nursing mothers might be complex. How much food is appropriate? What ought to be avoided? How might your baby's diet impact you? Observe these crucial dietary guidelines.

1) Giving your infant nourishment through nursing will support their growth and general health. However, you may be curious about the healthiest meals and beverages for you as

well as how your diet may affect your baby's development of breast milk.

2) Examining the particular dietary requirements of nursing moms is akin to setting out on a quest to provide for my child and myself. It's not just about what I eat; it's about realizing how my nutrition and my baby's growth interact in a complex dance.

3) See this investigation as a personal mission to shed light on the amazing physical changes that occur in my body as I nurse. Maintaining my health is not the only goal; it's also about giving my kid the best nourishment possible during this wonderful nursing journey, where my diet has a direct impact on their development and wellbeing.

We go further into the spotlight nutrition in this investigation. Imagine vitamin D taking the lead in enhancing our immunity as well as my bone health. Iron turns into my unsung hero, helping to meet our growing energy needs and standing by us both.

Think of this trip as an in-depth exploration of the world of B vitamins, the unsung heroes. They're not just about keeping us both mentally and physically fit right now; they're also very important in laying the groundwork for a long and healthy future.

Consider it a customized inquiry, understanding that my dietary requirements are as distinct as my fingerprint. Aspects like my age, way of life, and personal health are taken into account. It's about adjusting diet to meet the unique requirements of nursing while maintaining both my and my child's health.

In this investigation, staying hydrated becomes crucial. It is not only about the diet; it is also about drinking enough water to maintain milk production. Not only is it necessary to stay hydrated, but it's also a means for me to improve my general health and ease the transition to breastfeeding.

In the end, investigating the particular dietary requirements of nursing moms is an honoring of this remarkable stage in life. It's about arming myself with the knowledge I need to make decisions that support the joyful act of fostering new life in addition to providing nourishment for my body.

Do I require additional calories during nursing?
Indeed, you may require an extra 330 to 400 calories each day to provide you with the energy and nutrients required to make milk.

Choose nutrient-dense foods like a medium banana or apple, 8 ounces (227 grams) of yogurt, and a slice of whole-grain bread with a tablespoon (16 grams) of peanut butter to obtain these extra calories.

Which meals are appropriate to consume while nursing?
Making healthy decisions is your main priority to support your milk production. Choose foods high in protein, such as low-mercury seafood, lean meat, eggs, dairy, beans, and lentils. Pick a range of fruits and vegetables together with healthful grains.

The taste of your breast milk will vary if you eat a range of foods while nursing. This will introduce your child to a variety of flavors, which may make it easier for him or her to take solid foods in the future.

Your healthcare professional may suggest taking a daily multivitamin and mineral supplement until your baby is weaned in order to ensure that you and your child are getting all the vitamins you require.

How much water should I drink when nursing?
When you feel thirsty, sip on some water; if your pee has a dark yellow color, sip even more. Every time you breastfeed, you might have a glass of water or something else to drink.

Juices and sugary drinks, however, should be avoided. Consuming excessive amounts of sugar can hinder your attempts to shed pregnancy weight or cause weight gain. Caffeine excess can also be problematic. Don't consume more than two or three cups (16 or 24 ounces) of caffeinated beverages in a single day. Your infant may become agitated or have trouble sleeping if there is caffeine in your breast milk.

What about nursing when eating a vegetarian diet?

Selecting meals that will provide you with the necessary nutrients is especially crucial if you follow a vegetarian diet. As an illustration:

Select foods high in calcium, iron, and protein. Lentils, fortified cereals, leafy green vegetables, peas, and dried fruit like raisins are good sources of iron. Eat meals high in iron along with foods high in vitamin C, including citrus fruits, to aid your body's absorption of iron.

Think about plant-based sources of protein, like whole grains, legumes, nuts, seeds, and soy products and meat alternatives. Dairy and eggs are further alternatives.

Dark green vegetables and dairy products are good sources of calcium. Other possibilities include juices, cereals, soy milk, soy yogurt, and tofu, as well as goods that have been fortified and enhanced with calcium.

Which foods and beverages should I avoid or limit while nursing?

When nursing, you should use caution when consuming certain meals and beverages. As an illustration:

Booze: There is no alcohol content in breast milk that is deemed OK for a baby. If you drink, wait to nurse your baby until the alcohol has totally left your system. Depending on your body weight, this usually takes two to three hours for twelve ounces (355 milliliters) of 5% beer, five ounces (148 milliliters) of 11% wine, or 1.5 ounces (44 milliliters) of 40% liquor. Consider pumping milk to give your child later if you plan to drink alcohol beforehand.

Coffee: Limit your intake of caffeinated beverages to no more than two to three cups (16 to 24 ounces) each day. Your infant may become agitated or have trouble sleeping if there is caffeine in your breast milk.

Is my infant grumpy or is there an allergic reaction related to my diet?

Some foods or beverages in your diet may make your infant agitated or may trigger an allergic reaction in them. See your baby's doctor if, shortly after breastfeeding, your child starts to exhibit fussiness, develops a rash, diarrhea, or wheezing.

If you think your baby's behavior may be affected by something in your diet, try cutting out the food or drink for up to a week and seeing if it helps. Steer clear of foods like onions, garlic, and cabbage if possible.

Highlighting the contribution of postpartum vitamins to healing.

Your body doesn't instantly return to its pre-pregnancy state after giving delivery. While postnatal vitamins are just as vital for your overall health and well-being as prenatal vitamins are for the development of your unborn child. Any of a number of popular postnatal vitamins may be suggested by your healthcare professional to strengthen your immune system, aid in lactation, help with postpartum depression, and satisfy your nutritional needs.

Postnatal vitamins: what are they?

Any of a number of vitamins you take after giving birth is referred to as postnatal vitamin. They are critical for your own health as well as the health of your child, should you choose to breastfeed. Since babies need a lot of care and attention, it's simple to overlook your own health when making lists of things to accomplish. Postnatal vitamins can continue to fill in the nutritional deficiencies left by childbirth, as new mothers still require care.

New mothers may find it difficult to obtain certain essential nutrients, but a good postnatal multivitamin can help. Multivitamins are available for new parents who are unable or unable to breastfeed, as well as for lactating women and nursing moms.

Varieties of vitamins for postpartum

Prenatal and postnatal vitamins differ slightly from one another. Postnatal vitamins help with healing after delivery, whereas prenatal vitamins are designed to meet the nutritional needs of a developing infant. Furthermore, nursing mothers require much more additional nutrients than they did before becoming pregnant. Here are some essential ingredients for your supplement to replenish the vitamins lost during birth.

Magnesium, zinc, and calcium

Mothers who are nursing frequently do not consume enough calcium, zinc, or magnesium in their diets. Zinc helps strengthen your immune system when you're still susceptible from birth, coupled with vitamin C. Magnesium promotes overall healthy growth, whereas calcium assists the development of strong bones and muscles.

Iron

Anemia can occur in nursing moms who don't receive enough iron in their diet. Aiming for a daily iron intake of roughly 10 mg will assist boost energy levels and ease the transition of caring for a newborn. Your baby's red blood cells need iron to provide oxygen to the brain, but breast milk doesn't contain much of it. Rather, they can hold onto their iron reserves for up to six months before they require iron from their food.

D, A, and C vitamins

You might need to take a supplement if you don't get enough vitamin D from your diet or from spending time in the sun with your infant. Vitamin D is crucial for the development of your baby's bones. Your infant could have rickets, a condition where their bones begin to soften, if they don't get enough vitamin D. Additionally crucial to your baby's ability to absorb calcium and phosphorus is vitamin D.

Vitamin A is critical for the growth of the infant as well as for nursing mothers. Vitamin A supports good vision, tissue growth, and the immune system in both parents and infants.

In addition to strengthening your immune system to fend against future infections, vitamin C aids in the healing of your body from birth.

Chondroitinase, cholinergic acid, and iodide

During breastfeeding, there is an even greater demand for iodine and choline than there is for pregnant women. Iodide is critical for thyroid function, and it also aids in the development of your baby's brain and nervous system. For a year after giving birth, nursing parents should take 550 mg of choline and 290 mcg of iodine daily.

Docosahexaenoic acid, often known as DHA, is an omega-3 fatty acid that supports your baby's healthy development of the nervous system, eyes, and brain. Since our bodies aren't composed of omega-3s, you must eliminate all of them from your diet.

What advantages do postnatal vitamins offer?
Postnatal vitamins are best for nursing since they offer the widest range of advantages. You must be able to give your infant the nutrients they require for healthy development because they are virtually totally dependent on you for their nutritional intake. With the right nutrition, nursing moms can promote their baby's growth, brain and nerve development, and bone health.

Additionally, there are postnatal supplements that are beneficial but not meant for breastfeeding. Benefits of postnatal vitamins for moms include immune system stimulation and aiding in the body's healing after giving birth. Consuming the right nutrients is essential to leading a healthy life.

Adverse reactions to postnatal supplements
The most frequent adverse reaction to postnatal supplements is stomach problems. You might experience nausea, mild cramps, or an upset stomach in general. To help with symptoms, try taking your multivitamin with food. Consult your doctor about additional possibilities if that doesn't help. Seek emergency medical treatment if you have symptoms

of an allergic response, such as hives, swelling, rash, or trouble breathing.

Constipation can be brought on by iron supplements in particular, so be sure to drink lots of water, include fiber in your diet, and engage in some light exercise.

CHAPTER 2: Essential Nutrients and Their Benefits

For new mothers, eating healthily is usually of utmost importance during pregnancy; yet, after the baby is born, these eating habits may be neglected. Postpartum nutrition is crucial, but it doesn't always receive the attention it merits. Many mothers are shocked to hear that during the first few weeks after their recovery from childbirth, they require more nutrients than they did during their pregnancy, especially if they are also breastfeeding.

For the benefit of both you and your child, a well-balanced diet and attention to your nutritional intake throughout the postnatal period are essential. We understand that it's easier said than done, but with a newborn requiring your time, attention, and lots of cuddles, let's explore postpartum nutrition and our best advice to make it easier on you.

Any nutrients that were prioritized for your unborn child during pregnancy must be replenished by your body.

Along with providing the nutrients required for recovery from the energy expended during labor, you also need to take care of any further repair and healing. This is crucial for any surgical delivery, rips, or episiotomies, but it also applies to every woman who is pregnant.

The body has to work harder to create nutrition-rich milk while breastfeeding, which increases energy expenditure and nutrient requirements.

The need to safeguard your mental health – although there isn't a single element linked to mental health disorders in mothers, diet can serve as a means of self-care during the delicate period of becoming a mother.

Unfortunately, because of all of these extra demands on the body and the fact that we have less time than ever to take care of ourselves, nutritional deficiencies unfortunately tend to occur more quickly during this part of a woman's life! As a new mother's body tries to meet her baby's needs, she may become depleted of vital nutrients. Being a mother is a physically and psychologically taxing job, and nutritional inadequacies can lead to a myriad of issues that make it even more difficult to perform at your best during this fleeting phase of life. However, you can make sure your body is well-supported by making nutrition and self-care a priority as well as asking for assistance when needed.

For new mothers, eating healthily is usually of utmost importance during pregnancy; yet, after the baby is born, these eating habits may be neglected. Postpartum nutrition is crucial, but it doesn't always receive the attention it merits. Many mothers are shocked to hear that during the first few weeks after their recovery from childbirth, they require more nutrients than they did during their pregnancy, especially if they are also breastfeeding.

For the benefit of both you and your child, a well-balanced diet and attention to your nutritional intake throughout the postnatal period are essential. We understand that it's easier said than done, but with a newborn requiring your time, attention, and lots of cuddles, let's explore postpartum nutrition and our best advice to make it easier on you.

Take a moment to reflect on the experiences your body has had leading up to this moment, and feel awestruck. You not only developed and carried a foetus that had a brand-new organ (the placenta), but you also gained extra tissue and fluid to accommodate your tiny traveler. You also experienced labor and delivery, which is a huge full-body event. Your general sense of exhaustion and your low energy level may not come as a surprise.

This is a critical period for your body to receive nourishment for both your own health and, if you are nursing, the growth and development of your unborn child. A few advantages of eating healthily after giving birth include the following:

1) Any nutrients that were prioritized for your unborn child during pregnancy must be replenished by your body.
2) Along with providing the nutrients required for recovery from the energy expended during labor, you also need to take care of any further repair and healing. This is crucial for any surgical delivery, rips, or episiotomies, but it also applies to every woman who is pregnant.

3) The body has to work harder to create nutrition-rich milk while breastfeeding, which increases energy expenditure and nutrient requirements.

4) The need to safeguard your mental health – although there isn't a single element linked to mental health disorders in mothers, diet can serve as a means of self-care during the delicate period of becoming a mother.

5) Unfortunately, because of all of these extra demands on the body and the fact that we have less time than ever to take care of ourselves, nutritional deficiencies unfortunately tend to occur more quickly during this part of a woman's life! As a new mother's body tries to meet her baby's needs, she may become depleted of vital nutrients. Being a mother is a physically and psychologically taxing job, and nutritional inadequacies can lead to a myriad of issues that make it even more difficult to perform at your best during this fleeting phase of life. However, you can make sure your body is well-supported by making nutrition and self-care a priority as well as asking for assistance when needed.

After delivery, replenish and repair

Your recovery may be "nutrient expensive" depending on the sort of birth you had, but regardless of what transpired during labor, you still need to refuel and consume lots of extra nutrients to account for mending and any blood loss. Make sure you select the greatest supplements to support you when trying to improve your consumption of nutrients.

Even the "straightest-forward" births require a great deal of healing in the aftermath. Your uterus shrinks back down, your breasts adjust to the needs of your kid, your hormones rebalance, your skin and connective tissues restore suppleness, and that's just the tip of the iceberg when it comes to how your body changes and adapts.

Where there has been greater intervention during the birth e.g. Those who have a C-section or who are injured during a vaginal birth need a lot more food and energy to recover.

Which nutrients are beneficial for postpartum healing?

- Collagen
- Vitamin C
- Iron
- B12 vitamin
- folic acid
- magnesium

In terms of nutrition, the body needs a lot of protein for repairing tissues, particularly the amino acids proline and glycine, which aid in the production of collagen. Since collagen is essentially the "glue" that keeps the body strong, functional, and healthy, vitamin C is also required to support the body's production of collagen.

After giving birth, iron is frequently a focus because the process can frequently result in blood loss, which means you need to top off your stores. Eating a lot of iron-rich foods, such as meats, fish, lentils, spinach, and eggs, will help you do this. Once more, getting lots of vitamin C is essential as it promotes iron absorption and promotes wound healing.

Vitamin B12 is another "blood building nutrient" that is necessary for the synthesis of energy and for the formation of our DNA. It is hypothesized that infants who do not receive enough B12 are frequently more agitated and are more likely to not flourish. Seafood, eggs, liver, beef, salmon, and fortified milks are good sources of this vitamin. It is advised that vegetarians supplement with B12.

While folic acid is widely recognized for its significance in pregnancy, choline is just as crucial for memory and brain development. Breastfeeding mothers have the highest need for this vitamin. Eggs and organ meats, such as liver, are the best food sources of choline.

During the whole nursing process, magnesium supports your baby's growth and development. It's highly likely that your pregnancy has depleted your magnesium levels, thus supplementing with magnesium after birth is crucial. As a calming mineral, magnesium can also be enjoyed in the form of bath salts, which can be very helpful for calming the body and mind.

Nutrition that supports mood

Good fats and foods rich in fat-soluble nutrients, such vitamin A and E, help support hormone balance, which is crucial for healing. It is undeniable that during the initial weeks, your hormones require some (or a lot of) readjusting, thus it is a fantastic idea to prioritize foods like avocados, sweet potatoes, carrots, sunflower seeds, and almonds.

Our bodies give birth to a baby first during pregnancy, which means they lose a lot of brain-boosting nutrients like Omega 3. As a result, new moms are frequently deficient in this vital lipid. Studies have demonstrated the significance of Omega 3 in regulating our mood, averting postpartum depression, bolstering the immune system, and serving as the fundamental constituents of hormones. In addition to these advantages, maintaining high levels of Omega 3 guarantees that, if you are nursing, your milk will be of a high caliber and full of good fats. These necessary fatty acids are found in smaller levels in walnuts and flax seeds, but they are abundant in oily fish such as salmon, sardines, and mackerel.

Fortunately, vitamin D is a fat-soluble substance with a high profile that physicians and midwives frequently suggest. It not only supports the health of the brain, nervous system, and immune system, but it can also reduce the risk of anxiety and postpartum depression. Since sunlight provides the majority of our Vitamin D needs, taking supplements during the winter is advised. Even better, to make sure you are receiving the right dosage for your needs, have your vitamin D levels checked throughout the postpartum period.

Furthermore, breastfed moms should make sure they are getting enough vitamin D for their own needs as well as those of their unborn child, since newborns also acquire some vitamin D from their mother's milk.

During this period, particular minerals should also be the center of attention. In addition to iron, we also need calcium and zinc, which are included in cereals, green leafy vegetables, and high-quality animal products, to help us heal and restore our power. Particularly zinc is crucial for the immune system and postpartum recovery. In addition, it plays a significant role in hormone synthesis and has been demonstrated to benefit mental health, possibly mitigating postpartum depression symptoms. Assuring you are getting the appropriate quantity of protein at each meal is an excellent place to start because high-quality protein sources are frequently present in high concentrations of minerals. Whole grains, lentils, and beans are among other foods high in zinc.

examining the details of important nutrients such as iron, vitamin D, and B vitamins.

The contents of vitamins labeled as "postnatal" and "prenatal" are usually extremely comparable. Certain postnatal vitamins do, however, contain different amounts of nutrients that are especially meant for the body of a woman giving delivery. For example, some postnatal vitamins include extra iron to help with the body's recuperation after birth, extra vitamin D to aid in the body's absorption of calcium, and extra B vitamins to make sure nursing mothers and their infants get enough. In light of that,

Supplements Are Very Important if You're Nursing

It's likely insufficient for breastfeeding moms to obtain the essential nutrients required for their own and their child's best health from a well-balanced diet. For the length of breastfeeding, the World Health Organization advises nursing mothers to keep taking a prenatal vitamin. A baby's brain development, processing abilities, and visual acuity may benefit from continuing to take a prenatal or postnatal vitamin including folate, DHA, vitamin D, and iodine, according to one study.

It is crucial for parents to get enough vitamin D, but it is also critical for their children! Breast milk is insufficient in vitamin D for newborns on its own. As a result, until
they start eating solid foods, the American Academy of Pediatrics advises adding 400 IU of vitamin D daily to the diets of breastfed babies. Infant vitamin D drops are available at your local pharmacy.

For as long as they are breastfeeding, the CDC advises breastfeeding mothers who adhere to restrictive diets (such vegetarian or veganism) to take a prenatal or postnatal vitamin. A B12 deficiency can result from a diet low in animal proteins and induce symptoms in neonates such as anorexia, lethargy, delayed motor development, and blood issues.
Iron Is Vital

Any further justification for continuing postpartum prenatal vitamin use?
Elevated iron levels. The normal blood loss that occurs during labor makes it more crucial to restock iron stores throughout the fourth trimester. To make sure their iron levels are stable, moms can benefit from continuing to take prenatal or postnatal vitamins for three months after delivery, especially if they have a history of anemia. After this, if you're not breastfeeding, speak with your doctor to see whether you should keep taking prenatal or postnatal vitamins.

Pay Attention to Your Nutrition as Well

Try to eat healthily even if you're taking a vitamin after the baby is born. Giving your body the nourishment it needs to recover from its many hardships and maintain your new (and demanding) lifestyle as a mother is essential.

You can feel your best physically and mentally when you take care of your child by eating healthily and taking care of yourself. You can feel (even more) worn out, feeble, and psychologically depleted if you neglect your own health. As they say, "you can't pour from an empty cup!""

Even though the postpartum period is hazy and fitting meals in while taking care of a newborn can be challenging, try your hardest to focus on eating a balanced diet whenever you can. In particular, make sure you're receiving enough of the following after giving birth:

- Fish, lentils, and lean meats are good sources of protein.
- fiber found in fruits and vegetables
- Iron-rich foods include dark leafy greens, red meat, and legumes.
- Calcium found in foods such as beans, dairy, and dark greens
- foods high in folate, such as citrus fruits, leafy greens, and legumes
- foods high in omega-3 fatty acids, such as walnuts, seeds, and fatty fish

Presumptive mothers are often acquainted with prenatal supplements.

Prenatal vitamins, while similar to regular multivitamins, have additional folic acid to help prevent birth defects and frequently contain iron to support the increased blood volume associated with pregnancy, according to Dr. Jennifer Roelands, OB-GYN, chief medical officer at Well Woman MD, and fellow of the American Congress of Obstetricians and Gynecologists.

Iron, magnesium, and B vitamin shortages, however, are still very frequent after pregnancy and delivery;

according to Spare, these nutrient deficiencies are much more prevalent if you nurse or have two pregnancies that are close to one another.

Many of your postpartum nutritional needs can be met by taking leftover prenatal vitamins or even a typical multivitamin, but postnatal vitamins have extra advantages, according to Roelands. These advantages include increased levels of:

1) B vitamins contribute to energy production.
2) DHA, or docosahexaenoic acid, helps babies' brains develop if you breastfeed them.
3) Magnesium, which facilitates the relaxation of muscles.
4) Vitamin D and calcium are beneficial to nursing and brain function.
5) Fatty acids and selenium aid in the synthesis of hormones.
6) Because pregnancy puts a greater strain on your body's resources, eating a balanced diet alone won't always be adequate to prevent nutrient shortages. A postnatal vitamin should be taken in addition to a nutritious diet.

7) Breastfeeding is a beautiful but demanding journey. Your body changes dramatically as it replenishes its own resources and nurtures a new life. Proper nutrition becomes crucial to support this amazing feat. Vitamins D, iron, and B vitamins are important players in this nutritional orchestra, each with their own unique magic for mother and child.

Vitamin D: The Vitamin of Sunshine

Known as the "Sunshine Vitamin," a deficiency in Vitamin D can cause weakening of the bones and an increased risk of fractures. It is also vital for calcium absorption, which is necessary for the development of healthy bones and teeth in both mother and child.

Vitamin D Sources:

- **Sunlight exposure**: The main ingredient, 15 to 20 minutes in the midday sun can work miracles!
- **Fish that is high in fat:** Tuna, mackerel, and salmon are great options.

- **Foods fortified with nutrients:** Yogurt, milk, and cereals can all be beneficial.
- **Supplements:** If you don't get much sun exposure, see your doctor about the right dosage.

Iron: The Powerhouse of Oxygen

Anemia, exhaustion, and poor newborn development can result from an iron deficiency, which is particularly frequent during pregnancy and lactation. Iron transports oxygen throughout the body, which is essential for the synthesis of energy and red blood cells.

Iron Sources:

- **Red meat:** Iron is abundant in beef, lamb, and liver.
- **Poultry:** Turkey and chicken make excellent choices.
- **Seafood:** Iron powerhouses are oysters, clams, and mussels.
- Beans and lentils are great plant-based foods.
- **Foods fortified with iron:** Bread, pasta, and cereals can all make a big difference.

- **B Vitamins:** The Adaptable Enzymes
- The B vitamins are a vibrant group of eight that serve as coenzymes to support a variety of metabolic activities, including the synthesis of energy, the health of the neurological system, and the generation of red blood cells.

Here's a brief overview of several important B vitamins and where to find them:

Thiamine, or vitamin B1, can be found in whole grains, pork, and legumes.
Vitamin B2 (riboflavin): Found in leafy greens, dairy products, and eggs.
Niacin, or vitamin B3, can be found in fish, poultry, and peanuts.
Rich in bananas, chickpeas, and poultry is vitamin B6 (pyridoxine).
Rich in folate (vitamin B9) found in liver, lentils, and leafy greens.
Cobalamin, or vitamin B12, is mostly present in animal-based foods such dairy, meat, and shellfish.

Recall that it is essential to speak with your physician or a certified nutritionist to ascertain your specific requirements and the right dosages of any supplements, if any.

While these vitamins are important, it's important to keep in mind that the cornerstone for good nutrition during nursing is a balanced diet full of whole grains, fruits, vegetables, lean protein, and adequate amounts of water!

Being aware of how they affect immunity, energy, and general wellbeing.

Breastfeeding is a wonderful symphony of nurturing and nourishment, but it also puts a strain on your body, requiring a constant supply of essential nutrients. Of these nutrients, Vitamins D, Iron, and B vitamins are particularly important because of their individual functions as well as their combined effects on immunity, energy, and general health.

Sunshine for Your Soul (and Cells): Vitamin D Energy Booster: Sustaining stamina means bidding adieu to afternoon slumps and hello to optimal energy production, which keeps you feeling lively and prepared for those late-night feedings! Adequate Vitamin D levels help!

Immunity Guardian: Less sniffles and more smiles for you and your child as this vitamin of sunshine guards against infections and common illnesses!
Warrior for Well-Being: Low amounts of vitamin D can cause mood fluctuations and even depression. Keeping your levels at normal levels helps you feel balanced emotionally and invigorated.

..

Iron: The Transport of Oxygen:
- **Energy Engine:** Instead of leaving you feeling exhausted, consider iron as your own personal energy train, supplying power exactly where it's required. Iron transports oxygen throughout your body, supplying energy to every cell, including those that are working extra hours to produce milk.
- **Immunity Defender:** Adequate iron levels guarantee your immune system is well-equipped to fend off invaders, keeping you and your baby healthy. Oxygen is essential for immune cells to operate correctly.
- **Champion of Well-Being:** Low iron levels can lead to exhaustion, disorientation, and even hair loss. By maintaining enough iron levels, you can stay mentally and physically

healthy, feeling reenergized and prepared to take on motherhood.

- **B Complex Vitamins:** The Adaptable Band:
- **Energy Symphony:** No more mid-afternoon crashes—B vitamins keep the music going! B vitamins, such as B1, B2, and B6, are conductors in the orchestra that produce energy, guaranteeing effective fuel conversion and keeping you feeling motivated all day!
- **Immunity Harmony:** B vitamins are like harmony singers in your immune system, boosting your defenses and shielding your child from disease. They are essential for the creation of antibodies and immune cells.
- **Chorus of Well-Being:** B vitamins are vital for the neurological system, mood control, and cognitive health. Sufficient amounts support mental clarity, emotional stability, and general well-being, much like a happy chorus that lifts your soul.

Recall: The cornerstone of good nutrition during nursing is still a balanced diet full of fruits, vegetables, whole grains, and lean protein. During individualized advice on dietary tactics and possible supplement requirements, speak with your physician or a certified dietitian.

Remember, mama, you are the engine, the shield, and the conductor of your own health and happiness. Embrace the knowledge, nourish your body, and watch your inner power blossom along with your beautiful breastfeeding journey! By knowing the impact of Vitamins D, Iron, and B Vitamins on your energy, immunity, and overall well-being, you can make informed choices and fuel your breastfeeding journey with the power of good nutrition!

CHAPTER 3: Ailments and Natural Remedies

Transitioning into the postnatal period is like setting out on a personal adventure, when every day presents a different set of obstacles and successes. Let us delve into the complexities of these issues and discover the broad range of natural therapies that can act as gentle partners on this fascinating journey.

1. Challenge: Nurturing through Fatigue.Postnatal weariness, a familiar companion, is generally caused by interrupted sleep patterns and the physical demands of childbirth.

Natural remedies: Explore adaptogenic herbs like ashwagandha and rhodiola. They feel like delicate whispers of electricity to the body. Nurture yourself by eating nutrient-dense foods, staying hydrated, and including postnatal yoga to revive your core.

2. Embracing the emotional rollercoaster:

Challenge: Emotional upheaval, worry, and anxiety may accompany the transformative journey into parenthood.

Natural remedies: Immerse yourself in mindfulness and deep breathing techniques. Drink herbal teas flavored with chamomile or lavender for a soothing elixir for the spirit. Connecting with other mothers or seeking professional help becomes an essential component in managing mental well-being.

3. Exploring the Mysteries of Sleep:
Challenge: Irregular sleep patterns, which are common in the postnatal period, can have an impact on mood, energy, and overall well-being.

Natural remedies: Create a relaxing nighttime routine by including calming activities and disconnecting from electronics. For a relaxing night, try herbal drinks like valerian or passionflower. Don't underestimate the value of daytime naps for replenishing your sleep reservoir.

4. Dealing with the Shadows of Postpartum Depression:

Having the "baby blues" is a common sensation after giving birth to a child. Your hormone levels fluctuate after labor and delivery. These alterations can result in mood swings, anxiety, difficulty sleeping, and other symptoms. If your symptoms persist for more than two weeks, you may develop postpartum depression (PPD).

PPD affects around one out of every seven mothers after giving birth. It is typically far more acute than the early infant blues. You may have excessive crying spells. You may withdraw from friends, family, or other social situations. You might even think of hurting your child or yourself.
Additional symptoms include:

- Symptoms may include difficulty bonding with your infant and extreme mood changes.
- Symptoms include low energy, hostility, and irritation.
- difficulties making decisions.
- anxiety
- Panic attacks.

If you have these symptoms, tell your partner or a close friend. From there, you can schedule an appointment with your doctor to discuss treatment choices. PPD can linger for months if not treated, making it difficult to care for yourself and your infant.

Can natural therapies help?

After seeing your doctor, you may question if natural therapies can assist with your problems. There are options, but PPD is rarely treatable on its own. Inform your doctor about any medications you use as part of your holistic treatment plan.

Vitamins

Omega-3 fatty acids are receiving some interest from researchers as a potential treatment for PPD. In fact, a recent study found that a low dietary intake of omega-3s is connected with the onset of this type of depression. Though additional research is needed, nutritional reserves of omega-3 fatty acids are depleted significantly throughout pregnancy and after childbirth. Consider taking supplements and boosting your intake of meals like:

Options include flax seeds, chia seeds, salmon, sardines, and other oily fish.

Riboflavin, often known as vitamin B-2, may help reduce your risk of having PPD. In a study published in the Journal of Affective Disorders, researchers looked at this vitamin alongside folate, cobalamin, and pyridoxine. Riboflavin was the only one they discovered to have a favorable effect on mood disorders. The researchers recommend modest usage for best outcomes.

What else might I try?
Several lifestyle adjustments may help alleviate your symptoms:

Take care of your physique!
Consider taking long walks with your baby in a stroller or carrier. Purchase nutritious, whole foods at the grocery store. Sleep when you have the time, and take naps to fill the gaps. You should also avoid drinking and doing drugs.

Take time for yourself.
When you have a kid, it's easy to forget that you need time for yourself. Make it a practice to get dressed,

leave the house, and run an errand or see a friend alone.

Talk about it.

Avoid isolating yourself and keeping your emotions pent inside. Talk to your family, close friends, or spouse. If you don't feel at ease, consider attending a PPD support group. Your doctor may be able to refer you to some local resources. You can also join online groups.

Can treatment help?

Talk therapy is another excellent choice. It can allow you to discuss your ideas and feelings with a competent mental health professional. You can work with your therapist to develop objectives and discover solutions to the issues that are affecting you the most. Talking about your PPD may help you find more positive methods to deal with daily situations and issues.

You can try interpersonal therapy alone or in combination with drugs.

How is postpartum depression usually treated?

Antidepressants are commonly used to treat PPD. Your doctor may give tricyclic antidepressants (TCAs) or selective serotonin reuptake inhibitors (SSRIs).

If you are breastfeeding, consult with your doctor about the benefits and dangers of taking medicines. SSRIs, such as sertraline (Zoloft) and paroxetine (Paxil), are regarded as the safest options for breastfeeding moms, but they are still released in breast milk.

Some doctors may also recommend estrogen. Following childbirth, your estrogen levels decline rapidly, which may contribute to PPD. Your doctor may recommend that you wear an estrogen patch on your skin to assist boost your body's low levels of this hormone. Your doctor can also tell you whether this treatment is safe while breastfeeding.

PPD may resolve with treatment within six months. If you do not receive treatment or if you discontinue treatment prematurely, the illness may return or progress to chronic depression. The first step is to call out for assistance. Tell someone how you feel.

If you start treatment, don't stop until you're feeling better. It is critical to maintain open communication with your doctor and a strong support network.

5. Managing Breastfeeding Obstacles:
Challenge: Breastfeeding, while a beautiful relationship, can have drawbacks like engorgement, mastitis, and nipple discomfort.

Natural remedies: Cold compresses serve as calming companions for engorgement. Utilize the healing properties of herbal medicines like calendula or chamomile compresses. Seek advice on optimal latching technique to alleviate nipple discomfort.

6. Treating Aches and Pains:
Challenge: Postpartum joint and muscle ache is a result of the remarkable transformations your body has gone through.

Natural remedies: Take warm baths filled with Epsom salts. Experience the benefits of massages with arnica or lavender oil. Under the supervision of a healthcare expert, gradually incorporating postnatal activities can help to strengthen muscles and relieve pain.

CHAPTER 4: Fortifying Your Diet: Iron-Rich Recipes

Presenting a collection of easy and delicious recipes packed with iron

For a variety of reasons, women throughout their reproductive years need iron. In addition to promoting the production of red blood cells and immune system health, it also controls metabolism.

These dishes are meant to provide some extra flavor and nutrition to your postpartum experience. They're made with care to assist your healing and general well-being at this unique period, and they're tasty and straightforward. Have fun!

1. Recipe for Iron-Booster Smoothie

Duration: 5 minutes

You will need one cup of frozen mango.

One banana

2.3 cups of your preferred milk

Two TBSP of ground flaxseed

hefty bunch of kale

hefty bunch of spinach

Lemon juice squeeze

How to make it:

Put all the ingredients in a blender and process them until they are smooth.

Herb-infused tomato soup 2.

This reassuring classic can be more than just a childhood favorite of Americans.

You can turn an ordinary bowl of tomato soup into a soothing meal that supports your body's ability to manage inflammation and oxidative stress by adding fresh herbs and seasonings.

According to Swick, "one of the simplest ways we can increase the nutrient density in our diets is by using herbs and spices, which are truly nature's medicine."

She suggests attempting these to go with your soup:

- Basil, to lift your spirits (especially helpful for many new moms who could be suffering from postpartum depression, also called the "fourth-trimester blues").
- Parsley, since it aids in liver cleansing (and new mothers require a healthy detox, particularly as their bodies adjust to a new hormonal balance).

Due to its strong anti-inflammatory qualities and antibacterial qualities, turmeric is excellent for mending postpartum garlic.

3. Chicken soup, or caldo de pollo

The first forty days following childbirth are known in Mexican culture as the "cuarentena," during which the mother's only responsibilities are to relax, feed, and enjoy her new child.

The 40-day period was chosen because it is thought that it takes this long for a mother's reproductive organs to recover and return to their normal shape following childbirth.

Carrots and chicken soup, in whatever form, are frequently the permitted items to eat during the cuarentena. The choice of chicken soup is based on its reputation for being light and spicy—perfect for someone attempting to recuperate.

Since there isn't a particular chicken soup associated with the "cuarentena," I suggest tasting the homemade, traditional caldo de pollo. Carrots, tomatoes, garlic, lime, and safflower are included.

4. Bars of Chocolate Apricot

Time: two hours to relax and fifteen minutes to prepare.

Ingredients include peanut butter, dates, chopped dark chocolate, chopped almonds, rolled oats, chopped almonds, and salt.

Instructions:

In a food processor, pulse the apricots, dates, chocolate, and nuts until a crumbly, sticky mixture forms. Pulse in the peanut butter, sugar, and salt until smooth. Add oats and stir until well incorporated. Press into a parchment paper-lined baking tray or form into cookies.

5. Pie pockets with healthier chicken pot

Ingredients include cashew cream, veggies, chicken, and additional seasonings.

Instructions:

In a large pot, heat the oil over medium-low heat. When the onion is tender, add it and sauté it for a few minutes. Stir thoroughly after adding the garlic, ginger, and carrots. Curry paste is added. For three minutes, sauté. Pour in the coconut milk. Pour in a can of coconut milk (one and a half). Add the remaining ½ can of coconut milk to the pot after stirring in the cornstarch. Simmer after it boils. After coming to a boil, lower the heat and simmer the chicken and potatoes for 20 to 30 minutes, or until they are thoroughly cooked.

6. Oatmeal with Berries and Almonds Infused with Iron:

Add antioxidant-rich berries and iron-rich almonds to your morning oatmeal to make it better. Add some chia seeds on top for an added nutritional boost and the ideal way to start the day.

7. Curry with Sweet Potato and Chickpeas:

Cook sweet potatoes and chickpeas together in a delicious curry sauce. This filling recipe adds taste, warmth, and a healthy serving of iron to the postnatal table.

8.Delicious Chickpea and Potato Patties:

Chickpeas and sweet potatoes should be mashed before being shaped into patties and pan-fried till golden. These delicious patties are not only a brilliant method to increase your iron intake, but they also make a lovely dinner.

9. Chicken Breast Stuffed with Mushroom and Spinach:

Bake chicken breasts until they are perfectly done, stuffing them with sautéed mushrooms and spinach. This dish is packed full of protein and the spinach adds a healthy dose of iron.

10. Chocolate Banana Muffins with Iron Infusion:

For an additional iron boost, try baking some chocolate banana muffins with whole wheat flour. A guilt-free treat that both feeds and satisfies your sweet tooth.

These dishes are meant to provide some extra flavor and nutrition to your postpartum experience. They're made with care to assist your healing and general well-being at this unique period, and they're tasty and straightforward.

Addressing weariness with meals high in nutrients

The experience of becoming a mother throughout a pregnancy is nothing short of a wild trip. While there is a lot of information on pregnancy dos and don'ts and pregnancy is frequently celebrated, postpartum depression is not as well discussed. Maternity brings up a lot of emotions, which are difficult for them to understand or talk about.

A study published in the National Library of Medicine states that while the definition of postpartum fatigue has been defined rather widely, it usually refers to a diminished capacity for both physical and mental activity following childbirth, a chronic lack of energy, and difficulties paying attention and concentrating that are difficult to resolve with rest or sleep. To help with this, nutritionist Lovneet Batra recommended a few dietary adjustments. More energy is something that new mothers most frequently require.

Foods for Mothers to Eat to Reduce Stress After Giving Birth

In order to increase your postpartum energy and nourish and re energize yourself from the inside out, try these foods:

Moong Dal: Iron, potassium, copper, magnesium, fiber, vitamin B6, and folate are among the nutrients found in moong dal. B complex vitamins provide you with an energy boost and aid in the digestion of carbohydrates.

Almonds: Rich in fiber, healthy monounsaturated fats, and premium protein, almonds are an excellent food source. They include a wealth of B vitamins, which aid in the body's energy conversion from meals.

Roasted Pumpkin Seeds: Packed with fiber, healthy fats, and magnesium, pumpkin seeds are a great way to sustain energy levels.

Papaya: Rich in naturally occurring sugars like fructose, glucose, and sucrose, papayas are a tropical fruit that gives you a quick energy boost and are quickly absorbed by the body. Papayas also include enzymes including chymopapain and papain, which can promote better nutritional absorption and aid in digestion. This may improve the body's ability to absorb nutrients from diet and boost energy levels.

Ghee Adding ghee, a high source of omega 3, to your diet may help enhance your energy levels as fatigue is sometimes a sign of an underlying omega-3 shortage.

Processed foods and sugar: Use caution

Although there is no denying the appeal of a sugary treat, it frequently results in an energy spike that is quickly followed by a collapse. Maintaining a constant energy flow requires limiting added sugars and choosing entire, unprocessed foods. Maintaining vitality is more important than going on a sugar highs and lows rollercoaster.

Water

All physiological processes, including the healing process following childbirth, depend on water. It can aid with constipation prevention, edema reduction, and recovery time acceleration. Eight to ten glasses of water a day is the minimum, but if you're breastfeeding, try for more.

As long as you consistently use the restroom, water can help avoid bladder infections and replenish what is lost during milk production. Conversely, if you're not sure how much water is healthy for you, consult a dietitian or doctor. Drinking more water than normal can lower your blood sodium content.

In summary, water is necessary for survival and is crucial for healing after giving birth, particularly if you want to continue producing enough breast milk.

Another simple-to-digest meal that is ideal for new mothers is soup. It's simple to prepare ahead of time and nutrient-dense. When ready to eat, simply reheat!

Soup is easy to prepare ahead of time and ready for any occasion. It also helps replenish lost fluids and may be tailored to your specific nutritional needs. However, some people might find it insufficiently filling.

In summary, soup is a soothing and cozy choice that is easy on the stomach. To have leftovers for the rest of the week, make a large quantity.

Nut and Seed Laddoo:

Laddoos, as these delicious circular delights are called, are a sweet delicacy with several health advantages. These lactation laddoos are designed specifically to increase lactation in nursing moms by using a combination of nutrient-dense ingredients. They frequently include dried fruits, ghee, edible gum (gond), fennel seeds, fenugreek seeds, and garden cress seeds. In addition to satisfying your sweet craving, eating these laddoos gives you the vital nutrients you need for a speedy recovery after giving birth.

Dishes Made with Ginger:

Ginger can be a great addition to your postpartum meals to help with inflammation and digestion. Ginger may be a beneficial addition to your postpartum diet, encouraging general wellness, whether you choose to infuse it into your lentil soups (dals) or add it to your vegetables for enhanced flavor and health benefits.

Roasted vegetable and quinoa salad: a vibrant feast

Make a colorful quinoa salad with roasted veggies to nourish your health as well as your eyes. The roasted vegetables contribute a variety of nutrients, while the quinoa serves as a complete protein source. You can tailor this meal to your preferred seasonal vegetables and serve it for lunch or evening.

Activating Green Tea: An Increase in Liquid Antioxidants

Green tea stands out as an invigorating alternative when you think about your beverage options. With a modest caffeine level and a high antioxidant content, green tea gives you a little boost without making you feel jittery. Take a sip during your mid-afternoon break to give yourself a boost of energy.

Essentially, managing fatigue with nutrient-dense foods is a marathon of deliberate decisions rather than a sprint. It's about bringing a rainbow of nutrients into your day and crafting a culinary experience that awakens the spirit as well as nourishes the body. Thus, let every meal be an occasion to celebrate life, a self-care ritual, and a step toward becoming a more vibrant, energizing version of yourself.

CHAPTER 5: Brain-Boosting Recipes with Omega-3s

Exploring the importance of Omega-3 fatty acids, especially DHA.

The development of the brain is significantly influenced by omega-3 fatty acids. These fats also support blood coagulation, aid in immune system function, and facilitate the body's absorption of vitamins A, D, E, and K. Women who are expecting or who are already pregnant should maintain a balanced diet, which includes taking prenatal vitamins and prenatal Omega-3 supplements that include important fats, the most important of which are EPA and DHA, which are found in fish.

How long and when should I begin taking omega-3s?

A woman's supplement regimen should contain a pure, premium omega-3 fish oil before, throughout, and after pregnancy, as well as during breastfeeding. While EPA and DHA are both beneficial, DHA is more so throughout pregnancy and the first few months of a baby's life.

The reason these omega-3 fats are referred to as essential fats is that the body cannot produce them; instead, one must consume them through food or supplements. In addition to taking into account the fact that several pregnancies, particularly those that occur close together, might deplete the mother's store of omega-3 fatty acids, and DHA in particular, women should allow themselves at least six months before conception to build up this key necessary fat.

I can't just eat fish all the time.

The FDA advises women who are nursing, intend to become pregnant, or are currently pregnant to consume 8 to 12 ounces (2 to 3 servings) of mercury-free fish per week. The issue for women who are avoiding fish at the exact time when they most need DHA is that there is some concern about the presence of heavy metals, including mercury, in particular species of fish. Safe Catch tuna is recommended by the American Pregnancy Association because of its mercury testing process for every fish. Fish oil supplementation is a reliable method of getting EPA and DHA without risk.

How does DHA benefit my infant?

For the best possible development of the fetal brain, eye, immune system, and neurological system, DHA is necessary. It's crucial to take omega-3 fatty acids before being pregnant, but it's also critical to maintain enough amounts throughout the entire pregnancy. Due to its selective transference to the fetus, DHA levels in the mother gradually decline during pregnancy.

The greatest amount of brain growth occurs in the third trimester, and during this period, DHA is transmitted from the mother to the unborn child at an even faster rate. While this redistribution of DHA is necessary for the best possible development of the baby brain, eye, immune system, and nervous system, it can also deplete the mother's reserves and put her at risk for issues like postpartum depression that are linked to deficiencies in key fatty acids.

After delivery, is DHA really that important?

Indeed, a mother's DHA reserves can be transferred to the baby's breast milk through breastfeeding, thus her DHA levels may stay low after giving birth. Your newborn baby's brain continues to develop during the first two years of life, thus DHA is still essential during this period.

Infants born to moms with greater blood levels of DHA at delivery demonstrated advanced levels of attention spans far into their second year of life, according to University of Kansas researchers. These newborns outperformed babies whose mothers had lower DHA levels by two months during the first six months of life. John Colombo, Ph.D., the study's principal investigator, believes that early on in life, attentiveness is a crucial component of intelligence.

What else can my baby get from DHA?

Pregnant women who consume adequate DHA may see improvements in their unborn child's conduct, focus, and attention span. Having enough DHA during pregnancy has also been linked to improved immunological development and a lower risk of allergies in the fetus.

In children, lower brain DHA levels are linked to higher behavioral signs of anxiety, aggressiveness, and sadness as well as cognitive deficiencies. An excellent natural source of DHA for nursing mothers and expectant mothers is fish oil. Pregnant and nursing women should take 300–600 mg of DHA daily, according to international experts.

Make sure the fish oil you choose is of the highest caliber and has undergone meticulous processing to eliminate pollutants from the environment including dioxins, PCBs, and heavy metals. Research has shown that because fish oil can be treated to remove environmental contaminants, it may be a healthier source of DHA than seafood.

Keeping the Beat:

1. Heart Health

DHA and EPA work together to control the beat of your heart. This dynamic pair lowers the likelihood of irregular cardiac beats by keeping your heart pumping efficiently.

2. Controlling Fat:

DHA comes to your rescue if your triglyceride levels are producing problems. It resembles a firefighter extinguishing the flames of inflammation within your blood vessels.

Immunity and Inflammation:

1. Bringing Down Inflammation:

DHA is a whisperer of inflammation. It can tell when to "chill out, inflammation," which helps prevent the chronic form. It resembles the zen master in the field of fatty acids.

2. Increasing Defenses:

The immune system seems a little lethargic? DHA bolsters your immunological soldiers, enabling them to mount a defense against aggressors and maintain your health.

Discovering DHA in a Capsule and on Your Plate

1. From Ocean to Dinner Plate:

DHA hotspots are found in fatty fish like trout, salmon, and mackerel. Not only are these seafood treats delicious, but they're also a healthy way to meet your DHA needs.

2. Plant-Powered DHA: Supplemental Algal Oil:

Not a big fan of fish? Not an issue. Supplements containing algae-derived oil provide a plant-based substitute. It's like having the ocean on your plate without all the fishiness.

Omega-3s versus Omega-6s: A Balanced Act

It's important to keep everything harmonious. Although DHA has anti-inflammatory properties, an excess of Omega-6 fatty acids, which are present in processed foods, can also have an inflammatory effect. It all comes down to striking that perfect balance.

Final Thoughts: DHA: The Symphony Conductor of Your Body

DHA is the conductor of a symphony of immunological harmony, heart health, and brain brilliance in the grand concert of nourishment. Introducing DHA into your diet is like giving your body and mind front-row seats to a nourishing performance, whether it's in the shape of a seafood feast or a plant-powered pill.

Supplying recipes with foods high in Omega-3 to promote cognitive development.

Essential fats known as omega-3 fatty acids are critical for maintaining brain health and cognitive function. Consuming a diet high in foods high in omega-3 fatty acids can help maintain brain health, enhance memory, and possibly lower your risk of cognitive decline. The following are a few of the top foods high in omega-3 fatty acids that support cognitive function and brain health:

Salad with Salmon: Serve grilled salmon fillets on a bed of mixed greens. For a cool, omega-3-rich salad, add avocado, walnuts, and a lemon vinaigrette on top.

Chia Seed Pudding: Combine almond milk, vanilla essence, honey, and chia seeds. Put in the fridge for the night and garnish with fresh berries for a tasty breakfast or dessert that's high in omega-3s.

Crusted Chicken with Flaxseeds: Dust chicken breasts with ground flaxseeds and roast in the oven until crisp. For a well-balanced dinner, serve with steamed broccoli and a side of quinoa.

Sardine Toast: Spread whole-grain toast with mashed canned sardines and lemon juice. Add some sliced red onion and cucumbers to make a delicious open-faced sandwich.

Ingredients for the Coconut Chia Mango Smoothie:

- Chia seeds
- Milk from coconuts
- Diced Greek yogurt with mango
- Cubes of ice

Guidelines:

Chia seeds and coconut milk are blended until a gel-like consistency is achieved.

Add the ice cubes, mango dice, and creamy Greek yogurt. For a tropical smoothie full of Omega-3s that nourish the brain, blend until smooth.

Quinoa Salad with Smoked Salmon:

Components:

- cooked quinoa
- cured salmon
- Half a cherry tomato
- Diced cucumber and thinly sliced red onion
- new dill

Instructions: Combine chopped cucumber, cherry tomatoes, red onion, cooked quinoa, and smoked salmon.

To create a refreshing salad that is full of textures and brain-boosting Omega-3s, add some fresh dill and a little vinaigrette at the end.

Banana muffins with flaxseed: Ingredients:

- ripe bananas

- flour made from whole wheat
- meal made from flaxseed
- Greek yogurt
- Eggs with honey

Instructions: Mash ripe bananas and combine with eggs, Greek yogurt, honey, flaxseed meal, and whole wheat flour.

Bake into muffins for a delicious snack that combines flaxseeds' natural sweetness and their beneficial Omega-3 fatty acids.

Chicken breasts stuffed with spinach and feta cheese:

Ingredients

- fresh spinach
- Feta cheese
- minced garlic
- Olive oil
- Juice from lemons

Instructions: Stuff tasty mixture of crumbled feta and fresh spinach into butterfly chicken breasts.

Minced garlic is sautéed in olive oil until it turns yellow and is thoroughly cooked.

Serve with a squeeze of lemon for a delicious and cerebrally stimulating dinner.

Ingredients for Walnut-Crusted Baked Cod:

- Cod fillets
- broken walnuts
- Zest from lemons, garlic powder
- Olive oil
- Add pepper and salt.

Guidelines:

Coat the cod fillets with a blend of salt, pepper, garlic powder, crumbled walnuts, and zesty lemon.

Once the fish has a golden walnut coating and is flaky, drizzle it with olive oil and bake it. A crispy, high-Omega-3 treat.

Ingredients for the Salmon and Avocado Sushi Bowl:

- cooked quinoa
- sliced avocado, cubed fish, and fresh
- shredded seaweed nori
- cucumber with julienne
- Soy sauce

Guidelines:

Transfer the cooked quinoa into a bowl.

Add diced salmon, crisp cucumber, shredded nori, and creamy avocado slices on top.

Pour in some soy sauce to make a lovely bowl that's healthy and full of Omega-3s.

Chapter 6: B Vitamins and Daily Meal Planning

Simplifying the role of B Vitamins in maintaining energy levels.

B vitamins are essential for keeping the body's cells operating properly. They assist the body in converting food into energy (metabolism), producing new blood cells, and maintaining healthy skin, brain, and other tissues.

There are eight varieties of B vitamins, each with a specific function:

- Thiamin (vitamin B1)
- Riboflavin (vitamin B2)
- Niacin (vitamin B3)

- pantothenic acid (vitamin B 5)
- Vitamin B-6
- Biotin (vitamin B7)
- folate (vitamin B9)
- Vitamin B-12

Together, they are known as the vitamin B complex. The same foods frequently include B vitamins. Many people can obtain adequate B vitamins by consuming a range of nutrient-dense meals.

Those who struggle to achieve their basic demands, on the other hand, can benefit from supplements.

People may develop B vitamin deficiencies if they do not consume enough vitamins through their diet or supplements. They may also have a deficiency if their body is unable to absorb nutrients properly or if they are excreted in excess due to certain health conditions or medications.
Below, we will go over each B vitamin in greater detail.

Thiamine (vitamin B1)

The heart, liver, kidney, and brain are all high in thiamin. The body requires thiamine for:

- break down sugar (carbohydrate) molecules from food.
- Creating specific neurotransmitters (brain chemicals).
- Producing Fatty Acids
- synthesized certain hormones.

Foods containing thiamine

Thiamine is found in:
- Whole grains and fortified bread, cereal, pasta, and rice.
- Pork
- Trout
- Mussels
- Acorn squash
- Legumes, including black beans and soybeans.
- Seeds
- Nuts

Thiamine deficiency is uncommon in the United States. However, specific groups of people may not get enough thiamine, including:

- Those with alcohol dependence
- Older adults.
- Those with HIV or AIDS
- Those with diabetes
- Those with heart failure.
- Those who have undergone bariatric surgery

Symptoms of thiamine deficiency.
A person with thiamine deficiency may experience:

- Weight loss.
- Little or no appetite.
- Memory issues or confusion.
- Heart problems.
- Sensations of tingling and numbness in the hands and feet.
- Loss of muscle mass
- Poor reflexes

Alcoholism can lead to thiamine deficiency. This can lead to Wernicke-Korsakoff syndrome (WKS), which causes tingling and numbness in the hands and feet, as well as memory loss and confusion.

WKS can lead to Wernicke's encephalopathy (WE), a potentially fatal condition. A 2017 reviewTrusted Source discovered that people with WE may benefit from high doses of thiamine.

Riboflavin (vitamin B2)

Riboflavin is necessary for:

- Energy production
- Aiding the body in breaking down fats, drugs, and steroid hormones.
- Converting tryptophan to niacin (vitamin B-3).
- Converting vitamin B-6 into a coenzyme that the body requires.

Foods containing riboflavin

Foods high in riboflavin include:

- Organ meats
- Fortified breakfast cereals
- Oatmeal

- Yogurt and Milk
- Mushrooms
- Almonds

Symptoms of Riboflavin Deficiency

Riboflavin deficiency is uncommon, but it can occur when a person has an endocrine disorder, such as thyroid problems, or under certain conditions.

A person deficient in riboflavin may experience:

- Skin Disorders
- Sores in the corners of the mouth
- swelling of the mouth and throat.
- swollen, cracked lips
- Hair loss
- red, itchy eyes

Severe riboflavin shortage has been linked to cataract development and anemia. Pregnancy-related riboflavin deficiency increases the risk of several birth abnormalities.

The following people are most vulnerable to riboflavin deficiency:

- people who abstain from dairy products or who pursue a vegan diet
- meat-free athletes, particularly those who also abstain from dairy and other animal products
- ladies who are nursing or pregnant, particularly those who don't eat meat or dairy.

Niacin (vitamin B-3)

Niacin is transformed by the body into nicotinamide adenine dinucleotide (NAD), a coenzyme. The body uses NAD, the most vitamin-derived coenzyme, as a component of over 400 distinct enzyme processes. These enzymes help with:

- Converting the energy contained in carbohydrates, lipids, and proteins into a form that the Body can utilize
- Metabolic processes in the body's cells
- Communication among cells
- Expression of DNA in cells

Foods with niacin

Meat, chicken, and fish are examples of foods high in animal-based NAD that the body may readily utilize.

Nuts, legumes, and grains are examples of plant-based foods that provide niacin in a natural form that the body finds more difficult to utilize. Nonetheless, niacin is added by manufacturers to foods like cereals, and the body may readily utilize this form.

Symptoms of niacin deficiency
Getting too little niacin can cause a niacin deficiency. Severe niacin deficiency leads to pellagra, which may cause:

- Brown discoloration on skin exposed to sunlight
- Patches of skin with a rough appearance
- A bright red tongue
- Vomiting, diarrhea, or constipation
- Headache
- Fatigue
- Depression

Untreated pellagra can result in severe memory loss, behavioral abnormalities, and suicidal thoughts and actions. It might possibly result in death or a severe lack of appetite.

Individuals who may be at risk for a niacin shortage include those who:

- Malnutrition
- Anorexia nervosa
- Alcohol use disorder
- AIDS
- Inflammatory bowel disease (IBD)
- Hartnup disease
- Carcinoid syndrome, which results in the gastrointestinal tract developing tumors

Pantothenic acid (vitamin B-5)
The body needs pantothenic acid in order to produce new proteins, lipids, and coenzymes.

Pantothenic acid is a vitamin that red blood cells transport throughout the body, enabling many metabolic and energy-related functions.

Foods with pantothenic acid
Pantothenic acid can be found in many foods, however some of the foods with the highest concentrations include:

- Beef liver
- Shiitake mushrooms
- Sunflower seeds
- Chicken
- Tuna
- Avocados
- Fortified breakfast cereals

Symptoms of pantothenic acid deficiency
Pantothenic acid deficiency is rare in the U.S. because it is plentiful in many foods. However, it may affect people with severe malnutrition. In these situations, they typically lack additional nutrients as well.

Symptoms of deficiency include:

- Hands and feet burning and going numb
- Headache
- Irritability
- Restlessness and poor sleep
- A lack of appetite

People with a specific gene mutation called pantothenate kinase-associated neurodegeneration 2 mutation are at a high risk of deficiency.

Vitamin B-6

Pyridoxine, often known as vitamin B-6, is involved in over 100 different enzyme processes. The body needs vitamin B-6 for:

- Amino acid metabolism
- Breaking down carbohydrates and fats
- Brain development
- Immune function

Foods with vitamin B-6

The richest sources of vitamin B-6 include:

- Organ meats
- Chickpeas
- Tuna
- Salmon
- Poultry
- Potatoes
- Fortified cereals

Symptoms of vitamin B-6 deficiency

Many deficiencies in vitamin B-6 are linked to low levels of vitamin B-12, according to the National Institutes of Health (NIH) Office of Dietary SupplementsTrusted Source.

Vitamin B-6 deficiency may cause:

- anemia
- scaling on the lips
- cracks at corners of the mouth
- swollen tongue
- weakened immune system
- confusion
- depression

People at risk of a vitamin B-6 deficiency include those who have:

- Renal (kidney) disease
- Had a kidney transplant
- Celiac disease
- Crohn's disease
- Ulcerative colitis

- Autoimmune disorders such as rheumatoid arthritis
- Alcohol dependence

Biotin (vitamin B-7)

To a lot of supplements for skin, hair, and nails, manufacturers include biotin. However, the NIH state that there is not sufficient evidenceTrusted Source to conclude whether taking extra biotin helps with hair, skin, or nails.

Some individuals think that biotin could be beneficial for psoriasis.

The human body needs biotin for:
- Breaking down fats, carbohydrates, and protein
- Communication among cells in the body
- Regulation of DNA

Foods with biotin

Many foods contain biotin, including:

- Organ meats
- Eggs

- Salmon
- Pork
- Beef
- Sunflower seeds

Symptoms of biotin deficiency
Signs of a biotin deficiency include:

- Thinning of the hair
- A scaly rash surrounding the lips, nose, and eyes
- Brittle nails
- Depression
- Fatigue

Although deficiency is uncommon in the US, the following populations may be particularly vulnerable:

- Those suffering from a metabolic condition known as biotinidase deficiency
- People with alcohol use disorder
- Women who are pregnant or lactating

Folate (vitamin B-9)

The natural form of vitamin B-9 is called folate. Synthetic forms of the vitamin are found in fortified foods and some supplements, such as folic acid.

Because most people cannot take in enough leafy green vegetables for the levels needed in pregnancy, the Centers for Disease Control and Prevention (CDC)Trusted Source suggest that all women of reproductive age who wish to conceive take 400 mcg of folic acid each day, alongside eating a varied diet that contains folate.

When a woman has high enough levels of folate both before and during pregnancy, the fetus has a lower risk of certain birth defectsTrusted Source affecting the brain and spinal cord.

Folate is also essential for:

- DNA replication
- Metabolism of vitamins
- Metabolism of amino acids
- Proper cell division
- Foods with folate

The FDA requireTrusted Source manufacturers to add folic acid to standardized enriched grain products to help reduce the risk of neural tube defects. People can get folic acid from fortified breads and cereals.

Natural folate occurs in:

- Dark green leafy vegetables
- Beef liver
- Avocado
- Papaya
- Orange juice
- Eggs
- Beans
- Nuts

Symptoms of folate deficiency
Because folic acid is added to grain products, folate insufficiency is no longer frequent. On the other hand, the following are signs of a folate deficiency:

- Weakness
- Headache
- Heart palpitations
- Irritability

- Mouth or tongue sores
- Skin, hair, or nail changes

The FDA recommendTrusted Source that women increase the intake of folates and take folic acid supplements every day before becoming pregnant and
during pregnancy. Those in the following other categories may also require more folate:

- Alcohol use disorder
- Celiac disease
- Conditions that interfere with nutrient absorption
- IBD

Folic acid dosages exceeding 1,000 mcg per day are not recommended for humans. Taking more than this can mask symptoms of a vitamin B-12 deficiency Trusted Source. This can cause permanent nerve damage.

Vitamin B-12

Cobalt is a mineral found in vitamin B-12, which is frequently referred to as a "cobalamin." Vitamin B-12 is used by the body for:

- Creating new red blood cells
- DNA synthesis
- Brain and neurological function
- Fat and protein metabolism

Foods with vitamin B-12

Vitamin B-12 occurs naturally in animal products such as:

- Clams
- Beef liver
- Salmon
- Beef
- Milk and yogurt

It may be necessary for those who avoid animal products to obtain their vitamin B-12 from supplements or fortified foods like nutritional yeast and breakfast cereals.

Symptoms of vitamin B-12 deficiency

Vitamin B-12 deficiency usually causes a condition called megaloblastic anemia. Symptoms of a vitamin B-12 deficiency can include:

- Fatigue
- Weight loss.
- Constipation
- Loss of appetite
- Numbness and tingling in the hands and feet
- Memory problems
- Depression

Individuals who may be susceptible to a B-12 shortage comprise those who have:

- Circumstances that interfere with absorption of nutrients
- Older adults.
- Celiac disease
- Crohn's disease
- Undergone gastric bypass surgery or surgery on the stomach

Vegetarians, vegans, and women who are pregnant or nursing may also need extra vitamin B-12.

B vitamins each have their own unique activities, yet they depend upon one another for proper absorption and the optimum health advantages. Eating a healthful, diversified diet will generally give all the B vitamins a person needs.

People can cure and prevent B vitamin deficits by increasing their dietary consumption of high-vitamin foods or taking vitamin supplements.

Offering practical recommendations for adding B Vitamin-rich foods into everyday meals

Your body can't keep B vitamins for long, so they need to be supplemented periodically through your diet. Luckily, vitamin B foods generally include more than one B vitamin. For instance, numerous vitamin B6 foods, like salmon, chicken, and brown rice, are also strong providers of other B vitamins. If you don't have a digestive ailment or a limited diet,you're likely able to acquire enough of most B vitamins by eating a variety of meals each week.

The only situations when a dietician or physician could be concerned about particular vitamin B levels would be if you don't eat animal proteins or if you're going to become pregnant. Non-meat-eaters frequently need to hunt for fortified dietary options, like fortified cereal or tofu, to achieve the DV of B12.

Vitamin B-Rich Foods

To assist you add vitamin B foods in your diet, here is a list of the greatest sources.

Salmon

Salmon is highly high in B vitamins. Aside from the omega-3 fats, a 6-ounce fillet of salmon contains more than 200 percent of the DV for B12, approximately 100 percent of the DV for B3, 70 percent of the DV for B6, 42 percent of the DV for B5, 30 percent of the DV for B2, nearly 15 percent of the DV for B1, and 2 percent of the DV for B9.

Firm Tofu

According to Chow, tofu is a good plant-based source of B vitamins, albeit it may not be for everyone. A cup of raw, firm tofu contains 36% of the DV for B1, around 20% of the DV for B2 and B9, and nearly 15% of the DV for B6.

Tofu can also be fortified, making it an excellent source of B12 for vegetarians.

Green Peas
If you ate half a cup of peas for lunch and another half cup for dinner, you'd get 35% of the DV for B1, 25% of the DV for B9, and almost 20% of the DV for B2, B6, and B12.

Beef
Cooked beef is particularly high in B12, with around 4 micrograms per six-ounce serving (almost 190 percent of the DV). Aside from that, it contains approximately 75% of the DV for B2, 80% of the DV for B3, close to 50% of the DV for B6, and 25% of the DV for B5.

Avocado

If you want a creamy, savory side dish full in B vitamins, go no further than guacamole. One raw avocado has 30% of the DV for B6, 20% of the DV for B2, B3, and B9, and around 10% of the DV for B1.

Spinach

One cup of boiled spinach contains 262 micrograms of folic acid (66 percent of the daily value). Incorporating a cup of this dark, leafy green into your curry or pasta sauce gives 15% of the DV for B6, and 10% of the DV for B1 and B2.

Eggs

Eggs are high in vitamin B7, often known as biotin. A fried egg contains 25 micrograms of B7 (103 percent of the DV), 20% of the DV for B12 and B2, and 14% of the DV for B5.

Brown rice

In addition to the fiber, brown rice is a healthy carbohydrate that contains plenty of B vitamins. A cup of cooked brown rice provides 16 to 33 percent of the daily value for vitamins B1, B6, B3, and B5.

Another fantastic reason to make this grain a mainstay in your cuisine.

Chicken

Chicken is an excellent source of vitamin B6. A cooked 6-ounce portion of chicken breast contains 1 milligram of B6 (48 percent of the DV), 16 milligrams of B3 (100 percent of the DV), more than half of the DV for B5, about 30 percent of the DV for B2, and 15 percent of the DV for B1 and B12.

Lentils (and other legumes)

A cooked cup of lentils contains 90 percent of the daily value for vitamin B9, making it an excellent folate source for pregnant women following a plant-based diet. Lentils also contain more than 10% of the DV for vitamins B1, B5, and B6, as well as B3 and B2. Other legumes rich in vitamin B9 include edamame (green soy beans), pinto beans, and black beans.

Mushrooms

Mushrooms are an accessible source of vitamins B5, B3, and B2. One cup of sautéed white mushrooms contains 54% of the DV for B3, 32% of the DV for

B5, and 30% of the DV for B2. A three-ounce portion of fresh button mushrooms contains around 9 micrograms of vitamin B7, often known as biotin.

Asparagus

If you're planning a pregnancy and can tolerate asparagus, put it on your plate! A cup of cooked asparagus contains 67% of the DV for B9. You will also receive around 30% of the DV for B1, 20% of the DV for B2, and more than 10% of the DV for B3.

Chapter 7: Choosing the Right Postnatal Vitamin

A deep dive into selecting the most suitable postnatal vitamin supplement.

Pregnancy depletes several nutrients from the body. A postnatal supplement can help restore these critical vitamins and minerals.

Furthermore, maternal supplementation with postnatal vitamins is essential for breastfeeding moms, who require higher amounts of particular nutrients than during pregnancy. Breast milk production requires vitamin A, a complex of B vitamins, vitamin D, DHA, iodine, and choline.

Optimal nutrition, including dietary intake and postnatal supplements, is essential for a new mother to preserve her health throughout postpartum recovery while still having the energy to care for her infant.

How can I choose a good postnatal vitamin?
In addition to a healthy diet, a good postnatal supplement should contain all of the important vitamins and minerals found in whole foods. These include vitamin A, B vitamins, C, D, E, omega-3 fatty acids, calcium, iron, choline, folate, zinc oxide, magnesium oxide, and selenium.

An over-the-counter postnatal multivitamin may not provide all of the nutrients you require. Your doctor may recommend a postnatal vitamin as well as other nutritional supplements. The goal is to meet your specific nutritional requirements, as well as those of breastfeeding infants.

The correct postnatal care is especially vital for breastfeeding mothers. For example, if your postnatal supplement contains insufficient vitamin D, you may need to take an additional supplement. Alternatively, your doctor may offer iron-containing goods in addition to a postnatal vitamin to replace iron reserves, which are required for hemoglobin formation. One interesting feature about hemoglobin is that it aids red blood cells in delivering oxygen from the lungs to all body areas. Iron is necessary for babies' growth, particularly in the brain. Breastfeeding mothers may be advised to take a daily dose of docosahexaenoic acid (commonly abbreviated as DHA) to help their babies' growth and development.

Postnatal vitamins are typically started after giving delivery. Your doctor will advise you on when to start taking these postnatal supplements. The duration of your postnatal vitamin regimen is determined by your purpose for taking it. Some women continue to take a postnatal supplement until they discontinue breastfeeding. Others take a postnatal multivitamin to help them feel more like themselves before the pregnancy. Remember that mental health is just as essential as physical health; you shouldn't disregard the signs of "baby blues," and taking care of yourself will help you to give the greatest care to your new baby.

Your healthcare provider can advise you on when to discontinue postnatal supplements and move to a standard multivitamin for women.

Understanding labeling, formulas, and individual needs.

The Benefits of Reading Vitamin Labels and How to Do It

Do you ever look at the Nutrition Facts panel on foods at the grocery store? It's a terrific approach to ensure you're getting the nourishment you want and nothing you don't need. So you can do the same with vitamins! Dietary supplements are overseen by the Food and Drug Administration. The FDA defines a dietary supplement as a vitamin, mineral, herb, or other substance used in addition to food. It's a dietary supplement. And simply reading a product's label might reveal a lot about its ingredients.

First, check the benefits.

A dietary supplement label typically consists of a front panel, known as the Principal Display Panel, and a mandatory Supplement Facts panel. Begin by reading the front of the label. How will this product assist you? What are the main elements mentioned?

Does the formula align with your health goals? Does it align with your personal ideals, such as avoiding GMOs or buying more organic? You may wish to take various vitamins at different seasons of the year, particularly on workout or travel days. Understanding the benefits of each supplement will help you plan and alter your routine. You can consult with a healthcare practitioner to determine the finest supplements for you.

What is a Supplemental Facts Panel?
To learn more about the product, go to the Supplement Facts panel on the side or back of the container. This is fairly similar to the Nutrition Facts label that appears on food goods. Checking the Supplement Facts panel ensures that you are getting the most out of your supplements, including active components, serving size, and percentage Daily Value.

Components of Supplement Facts Panel
A Supplement Facts label, like a Nutrition Facts label, includes standard sections with crucial information. These sections are your buddies,

because they include a wealth of information to help you understand your supplement.

Serving Size and Ingredient Amount per Serving
The FDA labeling rules require firms to include the serving size, active substances, and measurable levels of components on the Supplement Facts panel. The serving size is the amount of product you would consume at one time—for example, one tablet. The amount per serving, indicated under serving size, represents how much of each component you receive in a single serving. These are measured using the standard unit for each ingredient. Amounts could be expressed as grams (g), milligrams (mg), or micrograms (mcg). Some substances are quantified in international units (IU), a measure of potency.

Active Ingredients
The elements mentioned just below "Amount per serving" are the active substances associated with the product's advantages. This list can help you learn important details about a component, such as its origin or processing method. For example, New Chapter's calcium is derived from a plant algae called Lithothamnion, as stated in the ingredients list. Our

riboflavin (a B vitamin) is fermented, as shown by the phrase "from ferment media" in the ingredients list. You can also learn about the plant parts utilized in herbal blends, such as the root, berry, or flower.

The Supplement Facts panel categorizes daily values into two categories: amount per serving and percentage daily value (%DV). The Food and Nutrition Board at the Institute of Medicine of the National Academies created Recommended Dietary Allowances (RDAs), which are used to calculate daily values. The recommended dietary intake for an ingredient may differ by age and gender. Daily Values, developed by the FDA, are frequently identical to the recommended dietary allowance for an ingredient and show how much of that ingredient is required daily. The % Daily Value represents the amount of that ingredient contained in each serving.You may observe that several supplement ingredients lack a percentage Daily Value. Herbs and mushrooms will be marked with an asterisk or a bullet in the %DV column. This is because only vitamins and minerals have specific suggested intakes.

Unless otherwise stated, the Daily Values are intended for adults and children aged four and up.

Other Ingredients.

Below the Supplement Facts panel, there is a section named "Other" or "Other Ingredients." These are elements that, while not considered active in the formula, are still necessary, such as the capsule itself. The list of "Other ingredients" is arranged by decreasing weight. For ease of reference, supplements would indicate any common allergies in bold below this section.

Additional Information

You may discover further information at the Supplement Facts panel.

Recommended Use

This is a crucial section that explains how to utilize the supplement, such as when to take it and if it should be taken with food. New Chapter® one-daily multivitamins, for example, can be taken on an empty stomach. If you have any questions or concerns about using supplements, consult with your doctor. It is not encouraged to utilize a vitamin or supplement for anything other than its intended purpose.

Expiration Date

The expiration date indicates how long your vitamin or supplement's efficacy is guaranteed. Vitamins and supplements can be expensive, therefore many individuals are concerned about the safety of taking them after the expiration date rather than discarding them. In general, it is not suggested to consume expired supplements. Harvard Medical School recommends storing vitamins and supplements in a cool, dry environment to extend their shelf life.

Cautions

Some labels provide cautions for customers with specific medical issues, while others merely urge you to contact your healthcare practitioner if you are taking any supplements. It is critical to read all cautions thoroughly. If you have any questions, ask your healthcare professional.

Certifications

Are gluten-free, vegan, organic, or non-GMO foods important to you? If so, check the package for third-party certifications! The NSF is a top third-party certifier of vitamins and supplements in the United States. Supplements are subjected to a range of tests to ensure their claims, product quality, and efficacy. Any NSF-certified vitamin or supplement will bear the NSF certification mark on the box or on the product's website. Other common validations are USDA Certified Organic and Non-GMO Project Verified.

Shop wisely!

We understand that with so many supplement options on the market today, it can be difficult to choose the correct one! That is why we advocate shopping wisely. Determine ahead of time what is important to you in supplements. Do you want your multivitamin to be vegetarian, organic, or GMO-free? How many tablets per day are you willing to take? Are you looking for a specific component or nutrient? Knowing the answers to these questions before going shopping will help you avoid confusion. The label and supplement facts panel has all of this information and more!

If you are shopping online and are unable to handle the container in your hands, check for photographs of the panels or a Supplement Facts list. Also, keep in mind that rules vary over time, and if a manufacturer updates a recipe, the supplement facts may alter as well. If you have any queries regarding a product, visit the manufacturer's website or call for assistance.

Finally, reviewing Supplement Facts labels can help you find the finest quality supplements that include everything you want and nothing you don't.

Chapter 8: Holistic Approaches to Wellness

Exploring self-care practices and their impact on postnatal health.

Some moms may get overwhelmed as they navigate motherhood, frequently prioritizing the needs of their families over their own. Self-care can have a substantial impact on one's mental, physical, and emotional well-being, driving some moms to seek a balance between their own and their children's health.

Learning how to use self-care effectively can be an important part of becoming the mother you want to be. There are various advantages to having this ability in your life, and you may be able to learn healthy coping techniques from a professional in treatment.

As a mother, you are not alone, and there is help available.

What is self-care, and why is it important?
Beyond the necessities for survival, humans can benefit from extra efforts to develop mental and physical well-being. The term "self-care" refers to any action that improves one's mental, physical, emotional, spiritual, or social wellbeing. Self-care can be beneficial since it allows you to focus on yourself rather than only external issues like your profession, family, or relationships.
The benefits of self-care for moms may include the following:

- A lower risk of future medical problems, such as heart disease

- More time to spend on developing and maintaining personal relationships.

- Improve your self-perception.

- Increased self-esteem

Self-care can help you maintain your mental health. Self-care helps you develop practical stress-management skills. If you suffer from sadness or anxiety, it can also help you lower the severity of your symptoms.

How would you describe a "good" mother?

While the definition of a healthy mother is subjective, several common traits and attributes that moms may possess can contribute to a more rewarding parenting experience.

Respect, tenderness, patience, empathy, support, healthy authoritativeness, and humility are often regarded as excellent qualities in a caregiver. Self-care can help you strike a balance and supply these and other traits to your family. Furthermore, children frequently emulate their parents, so seeing their mother practicing self-care can encourage them to choose to do the same for themselves.

Recognizing the symptoms of postpartum depression

Some moms may suffer profound sadness, disturbing thoughts, and other psychological problems following childbirth. While the "baby blues" are typical after childbirth and can continue for up to two weeks, other women have more severe symptoms. If you are feeling severe depression after giving birth or adopting a child, you may be suffering from peripartum depression, which starts during pregnancy, or postpartum depression.

The baby blues are not the same as postpartum depression, which usually requires medical attention from a therapist or psychiatrist. Understanding the common signs of postpartum depression and its possible manifestations can lead to shorter diagnostic processes, more effective treatment, and more happy experiences for both parents and children. Furthermore, postpartum depression is neither a weakness or a character flaw. Many people believe it is a complication of childbirth caused by an influx of hormones that might alter body and brain chemistry.

Everyone is susceptible to postpartum depression; mothers and people with gynecological reproductive systems are not the only ones. Fathers, adoptive parents, foster parents, and non-gestational partners may develop the disease after receiving a new child into their home. Self-care can help you detect the symptoms of a mental health illness early on, and getting therapy as a form of self-care can reduce the burden of postpartum depression on you and your loved ones.

Symptoms of Postpartum Depression
Postpartum depression is associated with a number of symptoms, such as the following:

- extreme mood fluctuations and low mood.
- Bonding with your new child is difficult.
- sleeping too much or not enough
- persistent thoughts of death or suicide
- The absence of enjoyment or interest in once-appreciated activities is known as anhedonia.
- extreme fear of becoming a "poor parent" or caregiver"

Why is self-care a problem for mothers?
Experts from the National Alliance on Mental Illness (NAMI) state that there are several reasons why people can find it difficult to put their own needs first.

For example, mothers may neglect to take proper care of themselves because they are too preoccupied with meeting the needs of their children.

It can be crucial to understand that parents are often the best caregivers for their children because they are also taking care of themselves. It could also help you to remember that self-care is not selfish and that you deserve to take the time to look after yourself.
Making self-care a priority might help you spend more time with your kids.
Think about setting both short- and long-term goals for your self-care practice when you first begin. After they've been recognized, you can create family-care strategies that help everyone emotionally connect or communicate well.

Remind yourself that self-care makes you the greatest version of yourself for your family, even when you may feel bad about leaving the kids with your partner to relax after a long day.

Try to change your perspective while you continue to take care of yourself by considering how you want your kids to handle their physical and mental health in the future.

An instruction manual on self-care.

For some people, learning to control your stress reactions is one of the most crucial components of self-care. By enabling you to let go of stress and strain in constructive ways as opposed to via self-denial, tension management can help you be a strong, caring influence in your family. You can attempt these self-care exercises.

Apply your senses.

There are several ways that sensory information from the five senses might assist you in managing stress. Playing with sensory toys, slime, or other materials can help you explore various channels and maintain a state of physical and mental relaxation. Some individuals apply a "worry stone," which is a smooth stone that they might touch with their finger to decompress during the day. Others use fidget toys, which have been demonstrated to be effective in reducing tension and anxiety.

Give yourself some time!

Set aside time to indulge in your hobbies without the presence of your partner or kids. You can better digest your day's emotions and get ready for potentially challenging circumstances by spending time alone. It might also give you a chance to relax and concentrate on your interests rather than what other people think of you.

Complete an item on your to-do list.
Mark off a task you've been putting off from your to-do list. It's normal to feel overwhelmed when you're overwhelmed with thoughts of what you "must do." It's possible that you envision these tasks as having more significance than the actual work. Once the task is finished, treat yourself to some downtime and a reduction in daydreaming.

Become the center of yourself.
Being centered means making connections with your environment, spirit, and values. Spending time outside, in prayer, or engaging in meditation might help some mothers develop this skill. At least once a week, engage in an activity that helps you feel a part of the world.

Concentrate on your basic needs.

A vital component of self-care might be meeting one's survival needs. Still, there are parents who find it difficult to exercise, sleep sufficiently, and eat healthily. Certain things can help you stay healthier, such as making a nightly routine, eating better meals, and going for regular walks. If being a parent makes it hard to find time for these interests, think about taking your kids along and turning it into a fun family activity, like going on a hike.

Maintain contact.

Continue to communicate with your social circle. In times of need, friends and family may be immensely supportive, inspiring, and motivating. People need social relationships for their mental and physical health, therefore try to build strong relationships with people, even if it means meeting other mothers at a parenting group.

Take into consideration several self-care methods.

For some women, being a "good mom" entails going above and above what they consider to be required. Contrarily, becoming a mother is a unique experience. It is often the case that treating your children with kindness, compassion, and generosity is a reflection of how you treat yourself. Consider the following alternate forms of self-care:

- Never evaluate yourself against others.
- Find out where your tension and sadness are coming from.
- Provide workable answers to your problems and put them into action.
- Seek assistance as required, both in your personal and professional life.
- Prioritize your own needs before attending to those of your children.

Recall that your kids do not possess a scorecard. Everyone is prone to error. If you make one, say you're sorry.

Check-in with your children and emphasize the value of self-care.

- Celebrate your successes.
- Talk to a therapist.

If you frequently undervalue your feelings, time, and well-being, consider seeking professional help and advice. Self-care can benefit from effort, emotional intelligence (recognizing and comprehending emotions), and literacy (communicating your thoughts, feelings, and needs), all of which can be learned with the help of a licensed therapist.

Working with a certified therapist online through a virtual therapy platform like BetterHelp can be a handy method for some mothers to integrate treatment into their hectic schedules, especially given the responsibilities of parenting. Online therapy, with its flexible appointment formats, frequently reduced charges, and shorter average wait times, can make treatment more accessible to people who previously had few options.

Some therapists employ online cognitive-behavioral therapy (CBT) to assist clients in identifying and changing harmful or maladaptive habits and thought patterns. A new study published in the American Journal of Psychiatry found that online CBT therapies can be just as beneficial as traditional face-to-face therapy. Online therapy can be more beneficial in some cases, particularly for people who have never attempted therapy before. Some clients find that therapy from home allows them to engage in more sessions.

It may be simpler to care for your children if you can also care for yourself. In this regard, self-care can be critical to your entire physical and emotional health. If you're having trouble developing a self-care regimen, consider reaching out to a professional online or in your neighborhood for further help and advice. You are not alone, and caring for oneself is frequently the first step toward caring for others.

Incorporating awareness and calm into daily activities.

Given their growing popularity, mindfulness practices such as meditation are being investigated in clinical trials to determine their usefulness in improving health outcomes throughout pregnancy and the postpartum period. We did a literature study to assemble and evaluate these research' findings. There is adequate evidence to support the use of mindfulness techniques during pregnancy to reduce anxiety, sadness, and stress, which may continue to have a positive impact after childbirth. There is limited data to support the advantages of mindfulness and meditation for other areas of pregnancy. However, given the low risk of these techniques, all women should be encouraged to practice mindfulness during pregnancy.

Mindfulness meditation has a number of emotional and physical health benefits for postpartum mothers that will last long after they give birth.
The benefits of practicing mindfulness during pregnancy are widely recognized, but they don't end there. Learning how to incorporate mindfulness into your everyday routine throughout the postpartum period and beyond is extremely beneficial to both your physical and mental wellbeing.

Mindfulness is a type of meditation that focuses on one's feelings and sensations in the present moment, without judgment or interpretation. BabyGaga just published an article about the benefits of practicing mindfulness while pregnant. Mindfulness has the ability to reduce stress and anxiety, increase mother-baby bonding and good development, avoid premature births, lessen the need for pain medication, and, most importantly, diminish the risk of postnatal depression. Mindfulness includes a variety of techniques designed to relax the user, such as breathing exercises and guided meditation.

However, attentiveness should not be abandoned after giving birth. Rather, to continue reaping the benefits of this type of mediation, it is necessary to practice it during and after the postpartum period.

Where to Begin?

1. Find a few minutes when you will not be distracted, such as when the baby is napping. You do not need to meditate for 30 minutes on the first day. Instead, start with five minutes and gradually increase the time over the course of many weeks.

2. Sit in a comfortable position that you can sustain. Traditionally, this is done cross-legged on the floor, but you can instead start on a chair. Make sure you can sit upright, relax your shoulders, and close your eyes.

3. After that, there are numerous techniques to meditate. Try a few of them to find what works

best for you. No matter whatever style you choose, remember that having a wandering mind is not a sign of failure; it simply indicates that you are human. If you notice your mind wandering, acknowledge it and gently return it to your area of focus.

4. Concentrate on your breath. Breathe deeply and evenly, possibly counting to five for each inhale and exhale.

5. Repeat a word or phrase. This is known as a mantra, and you might choose anything uplifting and positive that is relevant to you. You might even say "I love my daughter" or "I am a wonderful mom" repeatedly, either vocally or in your thinking. The objective is to focus on one word or phrase during the meditation.

The first time you try to meditate, you may feel overwhelmed since your mind refuses to calm down! Don't become discouraged. Everyone has a mind like that, and meditation is a technique. With enough time, your mind will learn to become quiet. In the meantime, you continue to profit from the practice.

According to Berkley University, approximately 15% of women in the United States who have given birth report experiencing postpartum depression, which is caused by a mix of hormones released after childbirth as well as the problems that come with having a newborn. A recent study conducted by the University of Wisconsin-Madison and UC San Francisco found that two days of mindfulness training can significantly improve a mother's labor experience and minimize her risk of PPD.

The study followed 30 pregnant, first-time moms in their third trimester who were thought to be at low risk of PPD. The participants and their birth partner attended a weekend-long childbirth education course. Throughout the retreat, half of the attendees attended a mindfulness session. In conclusion, the study discovered that mothers who attended the mindfulness portion had a better psychological experience with their labor than the other group that did not receive the same training. Similarly, they reported fewer levels of depression many weeks after having a baby.

When asked about the benefits of mindfulness for postpartum women and others, Donegan responded, "This is an area where the benefits are even more significant. Mindfulness meditation during pregnancy is connected with lower levels of prenatal and postpartum anxiety and depression. She continued, "As mothers, we are especially hard on ourselves and have high expectations." "When we fail to satisfy these expectations, we question ourselves and our ability as mothers. Mindful acceptance is critical during this time, especially when we are dealing with our new identity, lack of sleep, loss of control, and a changing body. We forget that we are learning on the job when we are not mentally or physically fit."

Mindfulness isn't just effective for preventing postpartum depression. It can also help to reduce postpartum discomfort. A 2017 study of 67 moms who had recently given birth discovered that mindfulness training was effective in lowering symptoms of postpartum depression in participants.

If you're dealing with your mental health after giving birth, whether or not you've been diagnosed with postpartum depression, mindfulness can help you get back on track. It is also preventive. For example, one study discovered that mindfulness-based cognitive treatment can protect people in remission from experiencing depressive symptoms; there was a 50% reduction in the likelihood of relapse within the first year after receiving mindfulness tools. According to the study's experts, this effectiveness rate exceeds that of antidepressant medication. Similarly, a separate study discovered that mindfulness can minimize the need for medical visits in persons who have a history of getting mental health care.

Many mothers experience mental health issues after giving birth, even if they are not formally diagnosed with PPD. Mindfulness is a simple way to improve your emotional well-being that requires only a few minutes every day. Getting into the habit of performing it on a regular basis can also assist your mental health in the long run, allowing you to maintain a happy mindset in order to prioritize yourself and your family.

Mental and physical health are equally vital, but you'll be pleased to know that mindfulness benefits both. According to Help Guide, regular mindfulness practice can help relieve stress, improve heart disease and gastrointestinal difficulties, lower blood pressure, lessen chronic pain, and enhance sleep.

According to Harvard University, a three-year-old study published in the Journal of the American Heart Association discovered that mindfulness meditation lowers the risk of heart disease. Mindfulness instills calmness in the body, which encourages the rest of the body to feel peaceful as well, lowering stress, blood pressure, and other indicators of heart disease.

That is not all. Mindfulness has been shown to help down cognitive loss caused by aging or Alzheimer's disease. A 2016 study of people with Alzheimer's disease, for example, discovered that participants who were assigned to the mindfulness mediation group had significantly higher cognitive scores than the other three groups, which tried cognitive stimulation therapy, relaxation training, or received no treatment. A 2017 study indicated that when adults practice mindfulness meditation on a regular basis, their attention span and focus improve.

According to Berkeley University, mindfulness has been related to improved immunological responses. "When we encounter viruses and other disease-causing organisms, our bodies send out troops of immune cells that circulate in the blood," according to the report. "These cells, which include pro- and anti-inflammatory proteins, neutrophils, T-cells, immunoglobulins, and natural killer cells, help us fight sickness and infection in a variety of ways. Mindfulness, it turns out, may influence these disease-fighting cells.

According to the magazine, research has shown that mindfulness can minimize cell aging. Cell ageing happens naturally as cells proliferate during a person's lifetime, but it can also be accelerated by disease or stress. However, research has shown that mindfulness has a favorable effect on proteins known as telomeres, which help combat the indications of aging. One study found that breast cancer survivors who exercised mindfulness were better able to retain the length of their telomeres than those who did not.

Chapter 9: Beyond Nutrition: Exercise and Well-being

Discussing the role of physical activity in postnatal recovery.

Regular exercise offers several health benefits, all of which apply to new mothers as well as later stages of life. These advantages include help with weight loss, improved cardio fitness, social engagement, and psychological well-being. Exercise after childbirth can also hasten recovery and help with muscular strength and tone.

Always ask your doctor or midwife before beginning any postnatal exercise regimen. It is recommended that you wait until your 6-week postnatal checkup with your doctor before beginning a group exercise program, returning to the gym, or receiving personal training. Individual circumstances, as well as postnatal issues, determine whether or not you are ready to exercise.

Benefits of Postnatal Exercise

- Exercising after having a baby can benefit your physical and mental health. It could:

- Exercise can enhance muscle strength and firmness, reduce fatigue, boost energy, and promote weight loss.
- Enhance cardiovascular fitness, strengthen abdominal muscles, reduce stress, and prevent postpartum depression.

When to begin postnatal exercises.
Gentle activity (like walking) can typically begin within a few days of giving birth, or as soon as you feel comfortable. Start when you're ready. Some ladies will feel able to begin exercising sooner.

Consult your doctor about the best time to restart an exercise regimen.

The majority of the alterations that occur during pregnancy will have reverted to normal within six weeks of birth. If you had a caesarean section, a difficult birth, or complications, it may take longer to feel ready to begin exercising. If you did not exercise while pregnant, begin with easy workouts and gradually progress to more difficult ones.

Keep in mind that your lower back and core abdominal muscles are weaker than they were before. Your ligaments and joints are also more supple and pliable, making it easier to harm yourself by stretching or twisting excessively. Avoid high-impact exercises or sports that involve frequent direction changes.

Breastfeeding and Exercise
Studies have indicated that strenuous or regular exercise has no negative impact on a mother's ability to properly breastfeed as long as fluid and caloric intake are maintained. Some study, however, suggests that high-intensity physical activity can

cause lactic acid to collect in breast milk, giving it a sour taste that a baby may dislike.

If you're breastfeeding, you can avoid this potential issue by engaging in low- to moderate-intensity physical activity and consuming lots of fluids before and after your workout.

The pelvic floor
Pregnancy and childbirth may have an unfavorable effect on the pelvic floor. Most women are taught pelvic floor exercises throughout pregnancy, which are vital to learn correctly and can be started soon after childbirth.

During pregnancy, the body undergoes hormonal alteration. Hormone levels begin to return to normal after birth, which for some women can cause mood swings, anxiety, irritation, and tears. Some women have postnatal depression, which is characterized by persistent low mood and irritability, negative thoughts, low energy, poor sleep, and, in some circumstances, difficulty caring for the newborn. Exercise improves mood and helps to maintain natural hormonal balance.

Postnatal exercise benefits all women; it not only helps to restore physical health, but it can also aid to improve low mood, sleep quality, stress relief, and the prevention of postnatal depression. Being fit and healthy also increases stamina, which helps the mother cope with the responsibilities of motherhood and makes caring for a newborn much simpler.

Presenting basic workouts appropriate for new mothers.

Types of Postnatal Exercise

Recommended postnatal exercises include:

1. For the first several weeks after birth, incorporate walking, pelvic floor exercises, and deep abdominal/core training.

2. After a 6-week check-up with a doctor or midwife, exercise with proper posture, light weights, and no breath holding. Swim once bleeding has stopped, then move on to water aerobics, yoga, pilates, or low-impact aerobic routines.

12-16 weeks postpartum

3. If the pelvic floor is optimised, it is possible to advance to higher impact activity such as jogging and sports, as well as increase load and volume. A physiotherapist who specializes in women's or pelvic health should assess this.

After 16 weeks postpartum

4. Increase the intensity of your exercise gradually, taking into account your pelvic

floor and abdominal levels, as well as any ongoing postnatal issues.

Consult your doctor or midwife for more recommendations and precautions.

Pelvic Floor Exercises
The pelvic floor muscles, located between the tailbone (coccyx) and the pubic bone, provide support for the colon, bladder, uterus (womb), and vagina. Childbirth can weaken these muscles, resulting in problems such as incontinence later in life.

1. To exercise them, first focus your attention on these muscles. To assist you identify these muscles, these are the ones you tense when you want to cease urinating. These exercises can be done sitting, lying down, or standing.

2. Try to relax your abdominal muscles. Don't hunker down or hold your breath. Squeeze and raise the tension gradually until the muscles are constricted as hard as possible. Release gently and slowly. Then, complete the exercises, which include:

3. Squeeze slowly, hold for 5–10 seconds, and then slowly release. Repeat ten times.
4. Make rapid, brief, and forceful squeezes. Repeat ten times.
5. Squeeze, then clear your throat or cough gently. Repeat three times.
6. Aim for 5–6 sets every day.

Making time for postnatal exercise.

Finding time to exercise while caring for a newborn might be difficult. Some days, you may simply be too weary to do a whole workout. However, this does not mean you should abandon physical activity. Do your best. Suggestions include:

1. Seek assistance from your partner, family, and friends.

2. Exercise with a friend to keep motivated.
3. Walking is an excellent approach to get back into shape; all you need is a pair of comfy sneakers. It's free and can be done practically anywhere, at any time.

4. While performing stomach exercises, include your baby by lying next to you on the floor.

5.

6. Exercising for 10 minutes at a time is OK. We understand that 150 minutes per week (as per the Physical activity and exercise guidelines for all Australians) seems like a lot of time, but you don't have to do it all at once. Not only is it better

7. to stretch your exercise out across the week, but you can also divide it into smaller pieces of time during the day.

Don't be too hard on yourself if your fitness plans fail. Just do your best, and know that you will have more time to yourself when your baby settles into a predictable schedule.

Tummy and pelvic floor exercises can be performed while completing other duties, whether seated or standing. To help you remember, try doing the exercises anytime you conduct certain activities, such as breastfeeding or driving.

For short travels, walk your infant in his or her stroller rather than driving.

Consider creating a home library of online exercise exercises. It may be beneficial to incorporate a few shorter workouts (such as 15 or 30 minutes) so that you do not constantly have to devote an hour or more to exercise.

General Exercise Safety Suggestions

Consult your doctor or midwife, but here are some broad suggestions:

1. Wear an appropriate bra that provides adequate support. Don't use your pre-pregnancy sports bra because your back and cup sizes are likely to have changed. Get measured for a new one.

2. Your exercises should not hurt. If you develop discomfort or other unexplained symptoms, stop exercising and see your doctor or a women's health physiotherapist.

3. Be mindful of postnatal depletion, which refers to symptoms caused by nutritional depletion, sleep loss, and significant changes in a new mother's role that might have an impact on your well-being.

   a. Warning signs: slow down.

Do not overexert yourself. If you exercise too hard, your body sends out warning signs, which can include:

Symptoms may include weariness, feeling ill, and muscle aches and strains.
Symptoms of postpartum vaginal flow include breast lumps or soreness, color changes to pink or red, and increased flow.
Lochia begins to flow again after it had stopped.

Chapter 10: Quick-Reference Guide

Condensing key information from each chapter into a user-friendly reference.

Assume you have a small pocket guide that summarizes the key topics from each chapter of "Postnatal Vitamins and Holistic Well Being." It's like a cheat sheet for navigating the postnatal period. Let's look at it.

1. Setting the Scene:
Prepare for the postnatal journey by focusing on general health and nutrition.

2. Holistic Vibes:
 - Understand the importance of balancing nutrition and health.

3. Nutrition 101:
 - Essential nutrients for postpartum health.

4. Breastfeeding Nutrition:
 - Learn about the unique nutritional requirements for breastfeeding mothers.

5. Essential Nutrients Unpacked:
 - Discover why Vitamin D, Iron, and B vitamins are your wellness superheroes.

6. Exploring the Specifics of Key Nutrients:
 - A closer look at Vitamin D, Iron, and B Vitamins and their benefits.

7. Powerhouse Nutrients:
 - How they support energy and immunity.

8. Nurturing nursing:
 - Linking nutrition and promoting nursing success.

9. Natural Remedies for Common Postnatal Struggles.

10. Recipes to Increase Iron and Reduce Fatigue: Quick and tasty dishes to help you stay motivated and overcome postpartum fatigue.

11. Omega-3 Benefits and Brain-Boosting Recipes:
 - Discover the benefits of Omega-3s and find recipes to increase your brainpower.

12. B Vitamins and Energy:
 - Learn about the benefits of B vitamins for maintaining energy levels.

13. Choosing the Right Supplement:
 - Tips for selecting the best postnatal vitamin for your individual needs.

14. Understanding Labels and Formulations:
 - Learn how to interpret labels and make informed choices.

15. Quick Recap:

- A concise overview to refresh your memory on the go.

Providing a convenient guide for busy mothers on the go.

Making a useful handbook suited for busy mothers on the go is similar to making a dependable companion that fits effortlessly into their hectic existence. Consider it a reliable partner, providing prompt and accessible assistance with the daily challenges of parenthood. Let's go into curating this valuable resource:

The Busy Mom's On-the-Go Guide: Navigating Life With Ease

1. Create a family calendar.
Having a single location where all family members' work schedules, appointments, commitments, and other comings and goings are recorded is critical for navigating the chaos of work and family life.

You'll know what you need to do that week at a glance, and it's a simple way to keep your caregiver informed about your family's routine, including the baby's.

Create a shared calendar on Google or with family organizer tools like Cozi or Hub, which you can access from your smartphone. You can also display a conventional wall calendar in the kitchen.

The calendar should include who will pick up your child and when, noting any changes, as well as any doctor's appointments, other commitments, day care closures, job obligations, and other family events.

2. Find good child care and have a positive relationship with your provider.
Find appropriate childcare and maintain a positive connection with your provider.

Finding decent child care, whether through a nanny, a large day care center, or a home day care, can help reduce some of the guilt and anguish associated with returning to work.

Whatever you decide, make sure to complete your research. Get referrals, investigate day care centers or nannies, conduct a walk-through if possible, verify references, inquire about immunization records, pay a surprise visit if possible, and have a backup sitter on hand.

It's also critical to talk frequently and openly with your nanny, babysitter, and/or day care teachers and administrators. This way, you'll be on top of your child's safety and well-being while still remaining actively involved in his daily life, which may help ease any guilt you feel about working.

If you opt to hire a nanny or sitter, you could request that she keep a daily log of the baby's schedule and development. That way, you will not miss anything! Even if you work from home, you won't always be "right there" to handle everything.

3. Divide and conquer.

If you have a spouse, sharing responsibilities can be really beneficial. Make sure you're both on the same page before your first day back at work. Coordinate your schedules and child care arrangements, and assign home responsibilities.

Make sure to prepare for sick days as well. If your infant becomes ill and/or requires medical attention, determine who will be in charge of caring for him or her.

4. Have a backup babysitter in place.

Even the most meticulously constructed strategies can fail. That is why it is prudent to have a backup sitter, family member, or close friend who can babysit in the event that your caregiver cancels, the daycare closes, or there is another emergency.

Another suggestion:
 Look for a fellow parent in the neighborhood who can help babysit for you in a pinch, and vice versa.

Make mornings as easy as possible.
Create a consistent morning routine for yourself, your baby, and other family members, and stick to it. That way, you'll know exactly what you need to complete before leaving for your commute or starting to work from home. And you won't waste much time bumbling around (but be realistic and flexible, because newborns, older children, and life in general are unpredictable!).

Try to perform part of your preparation the night before, such as packing lunches and snacks, making bottles, arranging everyone's clothes, having your baby's diaper bag ready, showering, and so on. Your mornings will run more smoothly if you rehearse and complete as much of your tasks ahead of time as possible.

Get the help you need at work.
Ensure that you have an open and honest relationship with your employer. Here are some ideas from experts:

Inquire about disease.
When you return to work, ask your employer or manager what their policy is for caring for sick children. Can you work from home (if you don't already)? Can you work on a flexible schedule? A similar question should be posed concerning your baby's doctor appointments. If you require two hours for a typical session, can you make up the time later?

Inquire about leave. Leave policies vary, so inquire about your employer's baby bonding policy, paternity leave policy, personal leave, sick leave, and unpaid leave.

Prepare to breastfeed.
If you're going to be pumping at work, dress comfortably so you can breastfeed without difficulty. Ask your employer about locations where you may pump comfortably and discretely, and attempt to establish a timetable so that your coworkers can

prepare for your time away from your desk. Also, when you return to work at the office, make sure there is a refrigerator where you can put your milk. According to federal legislation, every employer with 50 or more employees must give breastfeeding mothers an adequate break time during the day to pump milk for their newborns until the age of one. The company must also provide a private area other than the bathroom for pumping.

Get the infant to bed.
Establishing a consistent bedtime ritual is a terrific method to help your baby to fall asleep on time - something you'll learn to rely on at the end of a long day.

It's also worth noting that some babies don't sleep well during day care or with a sitter, which might result in overtiredness and/or more frequent night wakings.

Keep track of how much your baby sleeps each day. If your caregiver tells you that your child did not nap that day, try an earlier bedtime. A good night's sleep is essential for both of you.

Simplify dinner.

Who wants to spend time preparing dinner every night when there is a gorgeous infant to cuddle? When that little bundle grows into a toddler, what you make is no longer just for Mommy and Daddy, but also for your little one.

There are numerous strategies to optimize playtime while minimizing meal preparation time, allowing you to serve a nutritious dinner without putting in too much effort. Try these tips:

Plan your meals for the week.

Create a weekly menu. Plan your grocery list around the week's meals. Keep it simple, and swap out ingredients when you run out of something.

Prepare during the weekend.

If you're creating more elaborate meals, do so when you have more time, such as on the weekend or while the baby sleeps or naps. Make enough for at least a few meals, and freeze anything you won't eat immediately.

If you have a slow cooker, add the ingredients in the morning so that dinner is ready when you go home.

Prepare finger appetizers.

On days when you're too busy to prepare a meal, your children can still eat rather healthily. Prepare healthful finger meals such as crumbled hard-boiled eggs, cleaned and finely chopped, baby-safe fruits and vegetables, and little cheese cubes. For teeny tinies, try making purees ahead of time and freezing them in ice cube trays to defrost up when needed.

Take care of yourself!

This one can be difficult, especially when it seems like there aren't enough hours in the day. However, as much as you'd prefer to avoid taking care of yourself, your own health and well-being are critical to keeping everything running smoothly at home and at work.

If you can't picture taking time for yourself, try this to begin: Schedule at least one event for yourself each week while you're filling out the family calendar, such a pedicure, a weekend yoga session, a lunchtime haircut, or a shopping shop without the infant.

You'll be hooked once you've established the habit and seen how therapeutic and invigorating even a small amount of alone time can be.

Maintain a network of solid contacts.

Keeping in touch with your peers, coworkers, and job contacts takes time and effort (both of which you don't have much of these days), but there's a compelling reason it's worth adding to your already full to-do list.

Learn to say no.
Your time has never been more valuable. That is why you should spend your time doing what you need or want to do, rather than what others expect you to do.

Learning to say no is essential for getting everything done as a working parent. Time is a limited resource, and great parenting entails using it wisely. Here are some tips:

Be picky about your social calendar.
 Social commitments are most enjoyable when you have time to unwind. If that means saying, "Another

time, thanks!" to that friend's invitation so you can cuddle with your baby and get some rest, that's fine. The same applies for declining any volunteer opportunities until your schedule becomes more flexible. Being selfish with your time is something you should try not to feel bad about.

At the very least, many of those contacts may be working mothers like you who may offer advice, support, and commiseration when you're having a difficult week.

And you never know: If you find yourself exploring a different career opportunity, perhaps one with a more flexible schedule, those contacts could be really useful.

Outsource.
You don't need to do everything. It's okay to delegate and seek assistance when possible without feeling awful about it. If you have the resources and are comfortable with it, hire someone to clean your house, for example. Consider trying a prepared meal service. You can even employ someone to accomplish things you don't have time for, such as

going to the grocery store. Services such as Instacart will handle it for you.

Set reasonable expectations at work.

Saying no to professional obligations and requests can be even more tough, but setting expectations early on will help you feel less overwhelmed. If feasible, turn off your work computer at the end of the day so you may spend time with your infant without interruption.

Stay focused.

Many working parents discover that, despite having significantly more to do, they are more efficient and productive than before. The idea here is to stay focused and manage your time carefully.

Make a daily to-do list and stick to it, even if it means checking your email repeatedly or going to the store when you could order online. That way, you'll have more time to accomplish what you actually want to do: get things done so you can snuggle up with your gorgeous kid.

Sneak in some cuddling time.

Make time to cuddle with your baby, whether it's after a late-night feeding or an early-morning diaper change. Even though you might not be able to give your child your whole attention every day, try to make the most of the time you do have.

Balancing everything is a difficult task.
On days when you feel like you could give more at work or at home (or both), remind yourself that you're doing your best. Remember, you just delivered a beautiful life into the world, which is the greatest accomplishment of all.

Conclusion

Summarizing the holistic approach to postnatal well-being.

It's remarkable to bring a new life into the world, but it's crucial to keep in mind that the journey doesn't finish with delivery. In actuality, a mother's life is only getting started on a new chapter. The postpartum phase, which comes right after childbirth, requires tender care and attention.

For new mothers, the postpartum period is a sensitive and transformational time. For a smooth transition into parenthood, postpartum care entails physical healing, emotional support, and self-care techniques. Mothers can enter this new adventure with confidence and grace if they prioritize rest, nutrition, mental health, and urgent post-delivery care. Recall that the secret to a good postpartum period is to rely on a support system and ask medical professionals for advice and assistance.

Essentially, holistic postnatal care seeks to offer complete assistance in all these areas, acknowledging the interdependence of the physical, emotional, and social components of a new mother's life. It's a method that recognizes every mother is different and has particular demands throughout the postpartum phase.

Motivating moms to choose a healthy lifestyle for both themselves and their babies.

Starting a healthy diet is a journey that mothers and their priceless children take together. The decisions we make in the kitchen provide the groundwork for a prosperous life. Let's examine the typical obstacles and find easy fixes to care for mom and child together.

Moms frequently find it difficult to maintain a balanced diet for both themselves and their children because of the hectic nature of daily life. Confusion might result from juggling obligations, running out of time, and the deluge of information regarding what is actually healthy.

Maintaining a nutritious diet for mother and child is an investment in their lifetime well-being, not just what's on their plate. By tackling everyday problems with workable answers, we clear the path for a voyage full of life, development, and happiness.

Step one meal at a time, embark on this joint adventure, and watch as mom and baby's happiness and health grow.

Remember that the fundamental objective is growth, not perfection. To a healthy, happy, and full life!